30-MINUTE VEGAN COOKBOOK

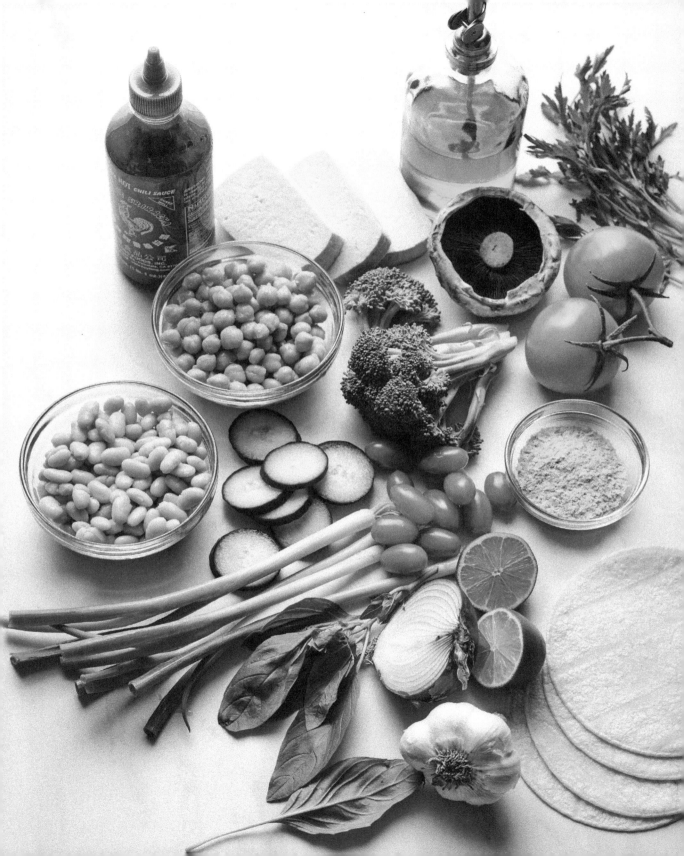

30-Minute
VEGAN
COOKBOOK

PLANT-BASED
FOOD IN A FLASH

ALLY LAZARE

PHOTOGRAPHY BY ANDREW PURCELL

ROCKRIDGE
PRESS

Interior and Cover Designer: Michael Cook
Art Producer: Sara Feinstein
Editor: Rachelle Cihonski
Production Editor: Nora Milman
Production Manager: Riley Hoffman

Photography © 2021 Andrew Purcell. Food styling by Carrie Purcell.

Cover: Tex-Mex Polenta Bowl

Paperback ISBN: 978-1-64876-748-7
eBook ISBN: 978-1-64876-749-4

R0

To my husband, Aaron, and my daughters,
Audrey and Autumn.
This book—and all the love
that went into it—is for you.

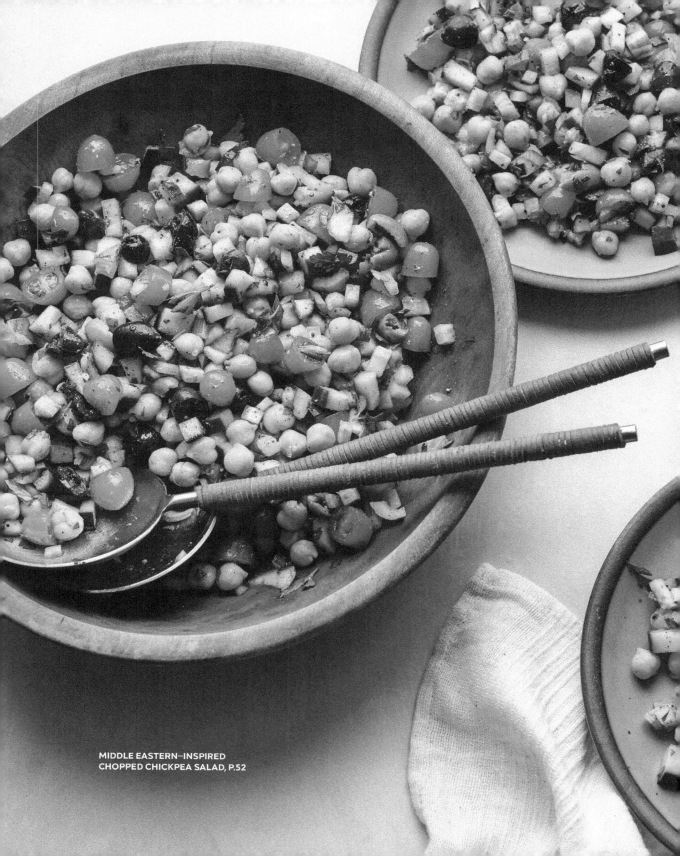

MIDDLE EASTERN–INSPIRED
CHOPPED CHICKPEA SALAD, P.52

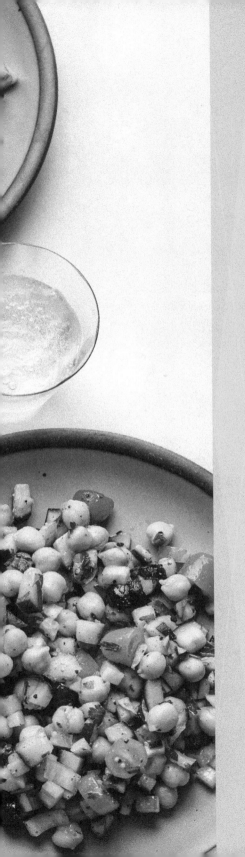

CONTENTS

Introduction   *viii*

1   Vegan Cooking in a Flash   *1*

2   Breakfasts & Brunches   *17*

3   Snacks & Bites   *29*

4   Soups, Salads & Sandwiches   *43*

5   Hearty Mains   *63*

6   Pasta & Noodles   *83*

7   Desserts   *103*

Measurement Conversions   *117*

Resources   *118*

Index   *120*

INTRODUCTION

Welcome to the *30-Minute Vegan Cookbook*. Chances are you're here because, like me, you're always looking for new and inspiring healthy vegan recipes that are packed full of flavor but don't take hours to make.

I love to cook, but being a busy mom of two small kids, I'm often pressed for time. I tend to fall into the rut of making the same thing over and over, or I reach for a takeout menu, which is rarely the healthiest option for our bodies—or our budget. They say necessity is the mother of invention, and my desire for delicious, easy vegan recipes that I can prep and serve in under half an hour led to the creation of this cookbook.

When we think of quick 30-minute meals, we often assume they involve using a lot of processed convenience foods rather than whole foods, which take longer to cook. The explosion of vegan convenience products available in mainstream supermarkets across North America suggests that we're relying on them more and more. I'll be the first to admit that products like plant-based meats and faux cheeses are handy to have, and from time to time they do appear in my recipes, but I'd like to dispel the myth that you must use them to create quick vegan meals. My goal with this book is to prove that you can eat a wide variety of delicious, flavor-packed vegan dishes that lean heavily on vegetables, beans, and grains, and don't have to include store-bought packaged processed proteins.

Throughout these pages, I'll show you how to maximize your shopping trips and stock your vegan kitchen, offer prep hacks to keep your daily kitchen time to a minimum, and give you recipes that push the boundaries of flavor and creativity, but still get dinner on the table in a hurry.

I've designed this book to be inclusive for everyone regardless of where they are on their plant-based journey, meaning you don't have to be a seasoned vegan to enjoy this book. Each chapter contains recipes that help everyone add a little more veg to their plates and appeal to every level of kitchen cook, from novice to expert. Experienced vegans will appreciate the diversity and creativity of recipes such as Jeweled Rice (page 66), Un-Crab Salad Po' Boy (page 60), Polenta-Stuffed Portobello Stacks (page 78), and Loaded Breakfast Sweet Potatoes (page 24).

If you're newer to the world of vegan eating, or you're veg-curious and want to find easy ways to include more vegetable-focused dishes in your diet, this book will give you easy, healthy, and delicious plant-based options for breakfasts, lunches, and dinners with recognizable ingredients and easy preparation methods, such as 15-Minute White Mac and "Cheese" with Broccoli (page 100), Black Bean and Sweet Potato Enchiladas (page 75), and Spicy Mixed Bean Jambalaya (page 80).

My goal for this book is to highlight just how easy it is to create 30-minute versions of popular and family-favorite dishes that follow the basic tenets of veganism (no animal products or by-products), and that focus on using real ingredients (with the occasional allowance for some store-bought conveniences, such as nondairy alternatives for items like milks and cheeses) and minimal salt, sugar, and oil. Life is about balance, and there is a way to successfully balance quick meal prep with healthy eating and convenience.

Vegan cooking doesn't have to be complicated, and vegetables paired with big, bold flavors can shine—even when you've only got 30 minutes to make dinner. So let's get cooking!

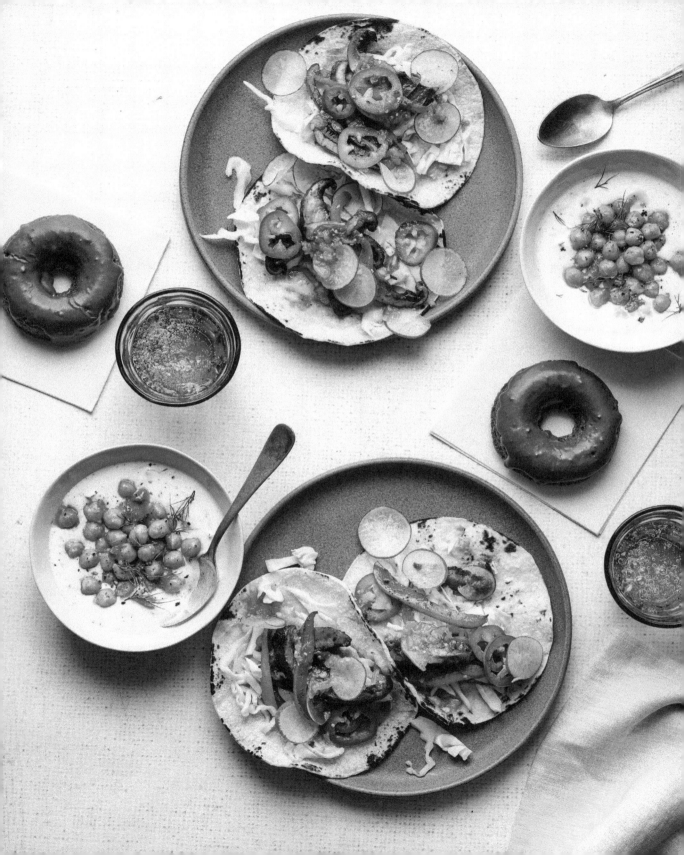

Vegan Cooking in a Flash

It's time to get started! Let's first talk about the benefits of 30-minute vegan cooking. Then we'll explore go-to ingredients, prep tips for time management, some must-have kitchen tools, and how to adapt recipes for people with specific dietary restrictions. We'll also cover how to swap out oil and salt without sacrificing flavor.

THE VEGAN LIFE

Mealtimes are important. They are a chance to start your morning off on a good note and to connect with your family while unwinding after a long day. And after a particularly tough day, there's nothing like a quick and delicious bowl of homemade comfort food.

For me, mealtimes are a chance to hang out with my family and have meaningful conversations. So I'm always looking for recipes that give me more table time and less "stressing over prep and cooking" time. That's why 30-minute meals are so great. I find that 30 minutes is long enough to put together a balanced meal (a main and a side dish, or a well-rounded one-pot meal) that everyone is going to enjoy without feeling like I'm trapped in the kitchen.

Getting balanced and delicious vegan meals on the table in a hurry can be challenging, though. After all, we don't have the supermarket rotisserie chicken to fall back on, and store-bought convenience foods rely on heavily processed ingredients that aren't always the most nutritious. Adopting a vegan diet means doing a lot of cooking from scratch, so having the tools and tips to shorten prep time, batch-cook ingredients, and multitask in the kitchen is key. That's where I come in.

Thirty-minute vegan meals aren't just for busy families like mine. The recipes I've included in this book are varied and unique enough to appeal to anyone looking for new and inspiring plant-based dishes. The techniques I use to get those meals on the table will inspire anyone who loves to cook but just doesn't have time, by taking everyday ingredients you likely have on hand (or can easily get) and adding lots of bold flavors to make mouthwatering recipes. After all, if a recipe is easy and uses ingredients you already have, you're more inclined to make it—even if you've never made a vegan meal before!

Simple, Healthy Ingredients

The best recipes are the ones that use ingredients you're familiar with and that are easily accessible. I've designed this book to focus on ingredients that are easy to find and store in your pantry or refrigerator and don't require hours of prep, like no-salt-added canned beans and legumes; quick-cooking grains like rice or quinoa; extra-firm tofu or tempeh; and frozen, canned, or prechopped vegetables.

When you're trying to cook a vegan meal in a short amount of time, it's easy to default to store-bought convenience foods. They are made to mimic the texture and flavor of omnivore proteins, and they often require very little prep. But there's a trade-off for that convenience in the form of salt, sugar, and fat.

Now, I'm not opposed to using oil, salt, and sugar (and even a few convenience products, like vegan butter) in moderation when I cook, but I'd prefer they be enhancers to healthy ingredients rather than the main ingredients themselves. There is truth in the saying that "fat is flavor," and I do believe it has a (relatively small) place in healthy vegan cooking. So having the option to use a bare minimum of oil to panfry jackfruit or tofu will add texture and flavor without tipping the scale on the healthiness of the dish.

Dietary Options

The main goal of this cookbook is to show you that delicious 30-minute vegan meals are possible—and that includes meals that follow other dietary restrictions as well. In addition to being vegan, many of the recipes I've created are (or can easily be adapted to be) gluten-, nut-, soy-, and even oil-free.

At the beginning of each recipe, I'll highlight whether it is free from common allergens like gluten, soy, or nuts, and where possible, I'll include a tip to easily convert that recipe to meet a specific dietary restriction, like swapping a whole-wheat pasta for gluten-free noodles, offering the choice of soy or almond milks for recipes, or choosing tamari or coconut aminos to eliminate soy and/or gluten.

Budget-Friendly

There are many ways to eat well-balanced, healthy vegan meals without breaking your budget. Eliminating the use of store-bought convenience foods is a great way to reduce your weekly grocery bills, as is shopping the sales. There is literally no difference between many brand-name and generic canned or frozen vegetables. The same goes for generic canned beans, legumes, and broths. So try adding them to your pantry—they are often much cheaper.

Another money-saving (and time-saving) tip is to buy shelf-stable grains, such as quinoa, brown rice, farro, barley, and others, in bulk and batch-cook them for the week. Make a double batch of your favorite grains on the weekend and store them in the refrigerator to use in a few different meals. Whole grains are inexpensive and can be worked into all kinds of dishes, and by having servings in the refrigerator that are ready to use, you'll have one less thing to prep for dinner at night.

Variety

It's easy to get stuck in a cooking rut or to think there's only so much you can do with vegan recipes. This book definitely challenges that theory and proves that variety is indeed the spice of life—and of vegan cooking!

Each chapter contains recipes that break the mold of what we think vegan food should be, or take familiar favorites and add an unexpected flavor twist—like savory Creamy Spinach and Mushroom Oatmeal (page 23) for breakfast; Green Goddess Dip Nachos (page 40) for the ultimate game night snack; and Everything Bagel Crusted Tofu Fillets and Green Beans (page 68) and Spicy Mixed Bean Jambalaya (page 80) for hearty dinners.

I'll show you how to use big, bold flavors and inspiration from global cuisines to give your meals variety, and incorporate an assortment of plant-based ingredients to add mouth-pleasing textures. Because vegan food is more than just salads and tofu.

✳ GOING OIL-FREE

While those who adopt a strictly whole-food plant-based diet will generally skip oils, many vegans choose to include healthy fats and oils in limited quantities. I tend to follow an "everything in moderation" philosophy with my cooking; therefore, many of the recipes in this book call for small amounts of light, neutral oil in the cooking process. I prefer grapeseed oil because it has a high smoke point, making it great for searing and caramelizing, and because a little really goes a long way, but you can use extra-virgin olive oil or even avocado oil. That being said, it is absolutely possible to create most of the dishes in this book without using oil. Sodium-free vegetable broth or even water are perfectly easy ways to quickly panfry vegetables and aromatics.

To water (or broth) sauté: Use a 2:1 ratio of liquid to oil (so a recipe that calls for 1 tablespoon of oil would need 2 tablespoons of water or broth instead), and lower your cooking temperature to medium instead of medium-high. The idea here is that by cooking low and slow, you can release the natural flavors and sugars in the vegetables that will allow them to soften and caramelize without adding fat. Never water sauté over high heat, and add more water or broth if needed to keep the vegetables from burning. This method will often take longer than cooking with oil, so be sure to factor that into your cook time.

A few recipes (less than 10) in this book call for the use of plant-based butter or margarine, and only when there wasn't a reasonable substitute that wouldn't drastically alter the success of the dish.

MASTER THE MINUTES

Thirty-minute meals are a great option for vegans because, for the most part, vegetables and soy-based proteins cook relatively quickly. But it still requires a certain amount of organization and preparation to keep your cooking time to that short half-hour window.

Half the dinnertime battle is figuring out what to make, scouring the cupboards and refrigerator for ingredients, and then getting to the prep and cooking part. By that point, most of us end up feeling frustrated and opt for the take-out menu drawer instead. Planning out your meals each week means it's just a matter of grabbing the ingredients and the pots or pans you're cooking with and turning on the stove or oven. Meal planning also helps manage your weekly grocery shopping by making sure you're shopping for all your ingredients at once, sticking to your budget, and not loading up on unhealthy convenience foods.

Prep Right

Learning how to maximize your prep time is another key element to ensuring you can get meals on the table in 30 minutes. Mastering even just a few basic kitchen skills can help elevate your prep game and keep you from spending half the night in the kitchen.

Cutting and Chopping

To maximize cooking time in these recipes, I've minimized the number of steps needed and tried to keep prep time to a maximum of 10 minutes, which is long enough to dice an onion and a couple of peppers, and peel and chop a carrot or potato. I've thought carefully about which vegetables are easiest to dice, which ones cook fastest, and which ones can be cooked along with something else to shorten prep (like adding broccoli or cauliflower florets to a pot of boiling pasta for the last few minutes of cooking).

For most of the recipes in this book, medium-diced vegetables will work just fine. They don't have to be perfectly cut, but attempting to keep them all relatively the same size will ensure they all finish cooking at the same time.

Measuring

In general, it's a good idea to use the proper tools to measure things that add salty, sweet, and hot flavors and liquids, as these are all ingredients that can adversely affect a dish if not measured correctly. Too much salt or cayenne pepper can make a dish unpleasant to eat, and too much liquid or too little can either drown or dry out your dish. So for ingredients like these, I do recommend using proper measuring cups and spoons for dry measures, and a good 4-cup measuring pitcher for liquids.

For other dry seasonings, sometimes it's faster to just eyeball it. If you're in a hurry, or you want to minimize the washing up after dinner, you can absolutely use your hands to measure out dry spices. Here's a quick guide to eyeballing dry seasonings.

- ► ⅛ teaspoon = one pinch between your thumb, index, and middle finger
- ► ¼ teaspoon = 2 pinches between your thumb, index, and middle finger
- ► ½ teaspoon = one US quarter-size amount in the palm of your hand
- ► 1 teaspoon = from the tip of your index finger to the first joint
- ► 1 tablespoon = size of your thumb

Precut and Premixed

One of the biggest keys to being a successful 30-minute cook is knowing where to take shortcuts that minimize prep time. For me, that's ensuring I'm not doing any busy work—fine dicing, mincing, and grating—unnecessarily.

For example, I recommend using jarred minced garlic where possible. Half a teaspoon is equal to one clove, but much faster to get in a pan. The same goes for fresh ginger. For all the dishes in this book that require fresh garlic or ginger, I've suggested using jarred versions, but I've also included the whole-food equivalent.

I'm also a huge fan of spice mixes. They are cheaper than buying each individual spice, take up less space in your pantry, require less measuring when cooking, and are handy for flavor profiles you use often. I recommend keeping the following five seasoning blends on hand to add bold punches of flavor in a flash.

- **Cajun seasoning**—A rustic, spicy mix of paprika (sweet and smoked), cayenne, garlic powder, black pepper, and oregano.
- **Curry powder**—A mix of turmeric, chili powder, coriander, cumin, ginger, and black pepper.
- **Everything bagel seasoning**—Dried onion, dried garlic, salt, poppy seeds, and black and white sesame seeds.
- **Italian seasoning (or pizza seasoning)**—A mix of classic Italian flavors: basil, oregano, marjoram, sage, thyme, and rosemary.
- **Taco or chili seasoning**—A flavorful mix of cumin, paprika, chili powder, oregano, garlic powder, onion powder, crushed red pepper flakes, and salt.

Time-Saving Cooking Strategies

Every good cook needs a few time-saving tricks up their sleeve. These are a few of the strategies I use to get good food on the table in a hurry.

Double-Duty Cooking

Need to steam some hearty veggies like broccoli or cauliflower, or want to cook a potato faster? Use the microwave to parcook them, which means quickly partially cooking them so that they soften, before adding them to your stovetop pan to finish cooking.

Another great trick is to use your boiling pasta water to cook hearty vegetables like carrots, broccoli, or cauliflower. Simply add them to the pot during the last 2 to 3 minutes of cooking, then strain with the pasta and add to your sauce.

You can also use your oven to help out here. Take advantage of the preheat time as actual cooking time. Unless you're baking a cake or making a complicated pastry like macarons, there's no need to wait for your oven to come to full temperature before cooking your food. Turn on your oven and pop your sheet pan of ingredients in there at the same time. Everything will start cooking as your oven heats up, shaving a few minutes off your overall cook time.

Buy Fresh and Frozen

Frozen vegetables are a 30-minute cook's best friend. Just about any vegetable is available in frozen form, including onions, and using them reduces your prep time drastically because they are already chopped (or sliced) and flash-frozen to seal in nutrients and minerals. Frozen vegetables are picked at their absolute ripest, so you're getting the full nutritional value without any of the prep work. Another added bonus is that they don't have to be thawed out first—you can cook them right from frozen.

Another great way to save time is to take advantage of your grocer's fresh precut veggie section. Making fajitas or tacos? Grab a package of sliced onions and peppers from the produce department. Feel like making a butternut squash soup but don't have time to peel and chop a whole squash? I guarantee your grocery store has bags or containers of precut squash all trimmed and ready to be added to a pot of boiling vegetable broth.

Make Ahead

All the meals in this book are designed to go from stovetop to table in 30 minutes, without having to prep additional components in advance. That being said, make-ahead ingredients are a great way to save time when you're rushing to get dinner on the table.

I like to batch-cook grains on the weekend and store them in the refrigerator for use during the week or freeze them in small freezer bags. Brown rice, quinoa, farro, barley, and even polenta freeze really well and are super simple to reheat when needed. If you're adding your frozen grain to a dish with sauce, it can go from freezer to cooking pan without defrosting. For grains being used without a sauce, like the Tex-Mex Polenta Bowl (page 72), place the frozen grains in a microwave-safe bowl with a tiny bit of water (about 2 tablespoons per serving) and microwave for 2 to 3 minutes, or until soft.

❄ DIETARY CONSIDERATIONS

My job here is to provide you with delicious meals that can be made in 30 minutes and that are easy to customize based on your preferences or dietary restrictions.

To make these recipes as healthy and as tasty as possible, I've leaned heavily on vegetables and avoided overusing processed foods like tofu and tempeh. (Tempeh is actually a less-processed and more gut-friendly plant-based protein and is a great swap for tofu, but it does take some getting used to!)

The only exception is the Pasta & Noodles chapter (page 83), but I've done my best there to suggest using fiber-rich whole-grain pastas and include recipes with rice- or vegetable-based noodles. And of course, you can always swap grain-based pasta for spiralized zucchini, carrot, or butternut squash noodles for an extra serving of veggies.

Each recipe includes nutritional information that breaks down (among other things) the calories, fat content, sodium levels, and protein in each dish so that you can make sure you're eating well based on your specific needs. While I did include some kosher salt throughout this book, I've done so knowing that the amounts suggested are small enough to add flavor without jeopardizing the healthiness of the dish. That being said, absolutely any recipe in this book can be made salt-free and still taste fantastic. Feel free to substitute your favorite salt-free seasoning for the kosher salt, or just omit it completely.

I've also added tags to each recipe to call out those that are nut-, soy-, or gluten-free for easy reference. As always though, use your best judgment based on what works for your diet and make the appropriate substitutions.

I have multiple food allergies, so I'm always reading labels carefully before using ingredients in my recipes. I encourage you to do the same if food allergies are an issue in your home. For readers with tree-nut allergies, the recipes in this book that are labeled nut-free may often include the use of coconut. While it is technically a fruit, the FDA has classified coconut as a tree nut, and because of this, you should speak with your doctor before using coconut in any recipe.

THE WELL-STOCKED VEGAN KITCHEN

A well-stocked kitchen is essential to successful 30-minute cooking. Most of the staple ingredients used in the recipes in this book are items you likely already have in your pantry. Here's a quick list of some of the foods I suggest keeping on hand at all times.

Ingredient Staples

Aromatics Jarred minced garlic and ginger, and aromatic pastes like tomato, curry, and fresh herb and chili pastes add intense, concentrated flavor to dishes with very little work. I also like to keep lemons, limes, and pure maple syrup on hand to add punches of sweet and sour flavor to dishes.

Bagged lettuce Bagged lettuces and lettuce or cabbage mixes are super handy for assembling a quick bowl. Add some veg, a protein like chickpeas or beans, some nuts or seeds for crunch, and a drizzle of tahini and you've got a delicious meal in less than 10 minutes.

Canned beans, legumes, and vegetables Chickpeas, beans, lentils, canned tomatoes, and even peas, corn, and carrots are great ways to quickly add flavor and protein to your dishes. Try to choose no-salt-added or low-sodium versions, and always rinse canned beans or legumes well before using.

Frozen vegetables and fruits Frozen vegetables and fruits are picked ripe and flash-frozen, ensuring that when you use them, you're getting the most nutrients possible. They are a great way to get a variety of flavors and colors into your meals with minimal prep work and are a great substitute for out-of-season fresh produce.

Nuts and seeds and their butters Pumpkin, sunflower, chia, and hemp seeds add great texture to bowls and salads, as do raw or dry-roasted almonds and cashews. Nut butters are great for adding flavor and richness to so many dishes and are great binders for no-bake desserts. Tahini (sesame seed paste) is the backbone of so many great sauces and dips, and a great whole-food substitute for nut butters.

Pastas and grains I like to keep a variety of quick-cooking grains on hand. Quinoa, couscous, pearl barley, basmati rice, and whole-grain pastas have long shelf lives and are usually ready in under 15 minutes.

Spice mixes Spice blends (see page 7) are great for adding tremendous flavor while taking up little space in your pantry. Dry spice mixes last about 6 months in the pantry. After that, they lose their flavor and should be replaced.

Tofu and tempeh Extra-firm tofu is my go-to for baking or panfrying because it naturally has more water removed from it and takes less time to press. Medium or soft tofu are great for replacing store-bought processed mayonnaise in sauces and dips, or in soups, like pho or ramen.

Vegetable broth There are always cartons of vegetable and mushroom broth in my pantry. Broths are the base for all soups and stews and are great way to pan-cook vegetables in oil-free diets. Choose no-salt-added or low-sodium versions if possible.

Tools and Equipment

I have a small kitchen, so counter and storage space are at a premium. I tend to choose equipment that can pull double duty or will get used daily.

Must-Have Kitchen Tools

These are the daily staples that you'll use over and over again to make the dishes in this book.

Blender If you're a smoothie fan, then an upright, high-speed blender would likely be a must in your kitchen. But if your blending needs are limited to soups, a less-expensive immersion or stick blender is a great tool to make easy work of pureeing soups. (If your budget and kitchen space allow, I recommend having both on hand!)

Box grater Box graters make quick work of shredding vegetables, tofu, and dairy-free cheeses. I have a box grater for heavy-duty work and a fine grater (also called a rasp grater) for zesting citrus.

Knives A good chef's knife and a smaller paring knife will get you through pretty much any kitchen prep task.

Large cutting board I prefer to use an 11-by-18-inch bamboo board that is solid enough to handle heavy-duty chopping and dicing.

Large skillet I love using an enameled cast-iron skillet. They last a lifetime and are so versatile (think stovetop to oven). A solid nonstick skillet works just as well for stovetop cooking.

Measuring cups and spoons You'll need a set of each, plus a measuring pitcher for liquids.

Metal colander or strainer Use it for straining pasta or rinsing and cleaning fruits and vegetables. Metal strainers also make great makeshift steamer baskets when set over a pot of boiling water.

Parchment paper or silicone mats For lining baking sheets; they make cleanup a breeze.

Pots and pans A large soup or stockpot for boiling pasta and making soup, and small and medium saucepans can get you through just about any stovetop cooking.

Spatulas, mixing spoons, and kitchen tongs Essential items for everyday mixing, cooking, and serving.

Standard-size rimmed baking sheets Aside from baking cookies, baking sheets are ideal for sheet pan dinners and for roasting tofu and veggies.

Vegetable peeler This is a necessary kitchen tool for making fast work of peeling vegetable skins.

If space and budget allow, the following tools are great optional items to help minimize prep.

- **Electric hand mixer** or **stand mixer**
- **Food processor** (8- or 12-cup)
- **Mandoline slicer** or small **electric food chopper**

Shopping and Planning

Successful vegan cooking involves being organized and prepared. Meal planning, keeping a stocked pantry and freezer, and regularly shopping for fresh vegetables are good ways to ensure you're never more than 30 minutes away from a well-balanced meal.

Grocery Shortcuts

Your best bet for maintaining a healthy vegan diet is to do most of your grocery shopping around the perimeter of the store. This means visiting the fresh produce section and the freezer section. Use the middle aisles only to get pantry staples like broth, rice and grains, and canned vegetables and legumes. As much as possible, try to avoid the vegan convenience foods section.

While faux meat and cheese products are easy and low-fuss, they are heavily processed products that rely on oils, salt, and fillers to bulk them up, and should be used in moderation.

Specialty Ingredients

For the most part, all of the ingredients in this book are items you'll find at a regular local grocery store. The exceptions are things like jackfruit, Korean rice cakes, and glass noodles, which are readily available at most Asian supermarkets, specialty grocery stores, and online, but are gaining popularity and becoming more widely available. Check your local grocery store for these items; you may be surprised to find them in stock!

ABOUT THE RECIPES

In this book you'll find recipes that are vibrant and full of flavor but still easily achievable in 30 minutes.

I believe life is about balance, and the recipes in this book reflect that philosophy. I've created dishes that rely first and foremost on using real foods, like vegetables, fruits, beans, and whole grains, such as whole grain pastas, rice, or bread. Occasionally, I'll call for the use of nondairy yogurts, plant-based milks, or other similar convenience products to add flavor and balance to the dish, while still making it as healthy as possible. To manage prep time and not overwhelm readers who may be new to vegan cooking, I've designed each recipe to include no more than 10 ingredients—excluding salt, pepper, and oil. Of course, you're welcome to add ingredients or swap out my choices for those that better suit your tastes, but the basic style of 10-ingredients-or-fewer cooking makes these recipes attainable while still unique enough to appeal to seasoned vegans looking for new inspiration.

I've sorted the recipes into chapters based on what type of meal you're looking for—breakfast, lunch, snack, or dinner. (There are two dinner chapters: Hearty Mains and Pasta & Noodles.) And yes, there's even a 30-minute dessert chapter—because everyone needs a little dessert now and then. Speaking of dessert, wherever possible, I've opted for natural sweeteners like maple syrup, agave, dates, or unsweetened applesauce. Occasionally a recipe may call for the use of actual sugar, in which case I recommend choosing organic coconut sugar instead of granulated white as much as possible.

Labels

Each recipe in this book is labeled to easily identify whether the recipe is suitable for any dietary restrictions you or your family may have, and to identify one-pot and freezer-friendly meals. You'll find the following labels throughout the book.

One-pot Recipes that use just one cooking vessel.

Freezer-friendly Recipes that freeze well, for days you don't have time or energy to cook.

Gluten-free Recipes that do not require the use of wheat- or other gluten-based products (if you do have a gluten allergy, always check ingredient packaging for gluten-free labeling to ensure that foods, especially oats, were processed in a completely gluten-free facility).

Nut-free Recipes that do not include peanuts or tree nuts (excluding coconut; see note in the "Dietary Considerations" box on page 9).

Oil-free Recipes that do not add any oil.

Soy-free Recipes that have no tofu or other soy products.

Tips

Throughout this chapter, I've included my go-to tips for shopping, prepping, storing, and cooking successful vegan dishes. In many of the recipes, I've also included tips to help you better prep or adapt a recipe.

You'll find the following tips throughout the book.

Cooking Tip Helpful information that makes the dish easier to prepare or cook, such as how to process a certain ingredient, or alternate cooking methods.

Ingredient Tip More information about a specific ingredient, including how to shop for, store, or use it, or alternate ways to use it.

Variation Tip Suggestions for swapping out ingredients to create a different version of the dish or substituting an ingredient to meet a dietary consideration.

✳ A NOTE ABOUT SALT AND OIL

All the recipes in this book can be made salt-free by choosing no-salt-added products and omitting or replacing kosher salt with a salt-free seasoning.

If you prefer to cook any of the recipes in this book without oil, follow the directions in the "Going Oil-Free" box (page 4) for a quick tutorial on water or broth sautéing. For recipes that require oil in a sauce, you can replace it with water or broth. For recipes that call for sesame oil (like the Tteokbokki on page 76), you can replace it with coconut aminos or even a teaspoon of tahini to add a toasted nutty flavor without adding oil.

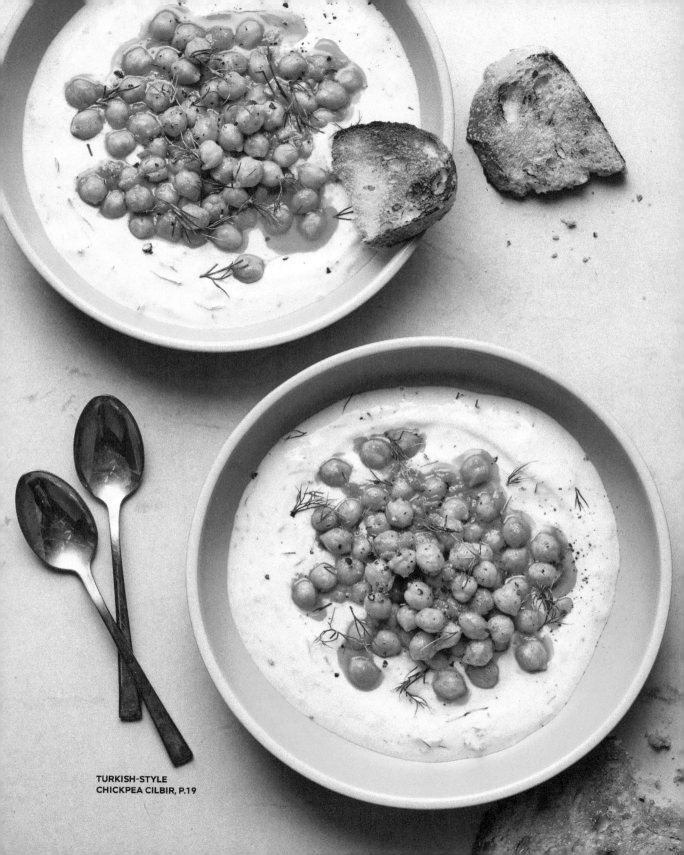

**TURKISH-STYLE
CHICKPEA CILBIR, P.19**

2

Breakfasts & Brunches

Maple Quinoa Fruit Salad 18

Turkish-Style Chickpea Cilbir 19

Sun-Dried Tomato and Zucchini Scones 20

Tomato and Almond Ricotta Toasts 21

Tempeh Hash-Stuffed Portobellos 22

Creamy Spinach and Mushroom Oatmeal 23

Loaded Breakfast Sweet Potatoes 24

Mixed Berry Breakfast Bread Pudding 25

Blueberry Lemon Pancakes 26

Chocolate Orange French Toast 27

Maple Quinoa Fruit Salad

SERVES 6   **PREP TIME:** 15 MINUTES   **COOK TIME:** 15 MINUTES
GLUTEN-FREE, NUT-FREE, OIL-FREE, SOY-FREE

Quinoa salad is a lunchtime staple for so many plant-based eaters, but this dish turns that concept on its side and showcases quinoa as a great breakfast choice. Quinoa is high in fiber and protein, and this fruit salad gives your morning a big energy boost. Sometimes I'll pair it with dairy-free strawberry yogurt for a delicious breakfast parfait.

1 cup uncooked quinoa

1 kiwi, peeled and diced

1 mango, diced

1½ cups sliced strawberries

1 cup raspberries

1 cup blackberries

¼ cup pure maple syrup

1 teaspoon lime zest

2 tablespoons lime juice

1. In a small pot, cook the quinoa according to the package directions. Drain, rinse under cold water, and drain again to stop the cooking process.

2. Meanwhile, in a large bowl, combine the kiwi, mango, strawberries, raspberries, and blackberries. Add the quinoa to the fruit.

3. In a small bowl, whisk together the maple syrup, lime zest, and lime juice. Pour over the fruit and quinoa and toss to coat before serving.

Cooking Tip: Since mornings can often be rushed, I find that sometimes it's easier to use pre-chopped fresh fruit or frozen fruit that I've thawed in the refrigerator overnight or rinsed under cool water for a few minutes first.

Per Serving: Calories: 223; Fat: 3g; Carbohydrates: 47g; Fiber: 7g; Sugar: 23g; Protein: 5g; Sodium: 7mg

Turkish-Style Chickpea Cilbir

SERVES 4 **PREP TIME:** 10 MINUTES **COOK TIME:** 10 MINUTES
NUT-FREE, SOY-FREE

Cilbir is a Turkish dish that dates back to the 15th century. Traditionally, it's made with poached eggs nestled in a garlic-infused yogurt, topped with a spicy butter sauce and served with bread to dip or scoop with. In this version, I've swapped the eggs for protein-packed chickpeas that are quickly panfried in spicy vegan butter, then nestled into a garlic-dill dairy-free yogurt (I like to use Daiya Greek plain coconut yogurt) and served with a sourdough slice for dipping.

2 cups dairy-free plain Greek yogurt

1 teaspoon jarred minced garlic or 2 garlic cloves, minced

2 tablespoons finely chopped fresh dill or 1 tablespoon dried dill

½ teaspoon kosher salt

½ teaspoon freshly ground black pepper

Juice of ½ lime

3 tablespoons vegan butter

½ teaspoon hot paprika, chili oil, or hot red pepper paste, plus more as needed

1 teaspoon sweet paprika

1 (15-ounce) can no-salt-added chickpeas, drained and rinsed

3 slices sourdough bread, halved lengthwise

1. In a large bowl, combine the yogurt, garlic, dill, salt, pepper, and lime juice. Stir and set aside.

2. In a medium skillet, combine the butter and hot and sweet paprikas. Cook over medium-high heat for 2 minutes, or until the butter just starts to bubble. Add the chickpeas and cook, stirring constantly, for 5 minutes, or until heated through. Remove from the heat and set aside.

3. Divide the yogurt into four bowls or rimmed plates. Top with the chickpeas and serve with sourdough bread for dipping.

Per Serving: Calories: 312; Fat: 15g; Carbohydrates: 35g; Fiber: 6g; Sugar: 5g; Protein: 10g; Sodium: 541mg

Sun-Dried Tomato and Zucchini Scones

MAKES 8 TO 10 SCONES   PREP TIME: 10 MINUTES   **COOK TIME:** 20 MINUTES
NUT-FREE

Years ago I perfected a vegan scone recipe, and since then I've enjoyed coming up with different flavor variations like sun-dried tomato and zucchini. I enjoy serving them for brunch as an alternative to bagels. If you're a fan of cheese scones and don't mind using vegan cheese shreds, try adding a half cup of vegan Cheddar or Monterey Jack shreds to the dough before baking.

2½ cups all-purpose flour

1 tablespoon baking powder

¼ cup nutritional yeast

1 teaspoon kosher salt

½ cup vegan butter, cold

¾ cup shredded zucchini, squeezed to remove water

6 oil-packed sun-dried tomatoes, patted dry and finely chopped

2 tablespoons minced fresh basil or 2 teaspoons dried basil

1 cup plain unsweetened soy milk

1. Preheat the oven to 425°F. Line a standard baking sheet with parchment paper and set aside.

2. In a large bowl, combine the flour, baking powder, nutritional yeast, and salt. Using a pastry cutter or two knives and working in a crisscross motion, cut the butter into the flour mix until it resembles coarse cornmeal. Stir in the zucchini, sun-dried tomatoes, and basil. Add the soy milk and stir just until a dough forms.

3. Using a ⅓-cup measure, drop balls of dough onto the prepared baking sheet, spacing them about 2 inches apart. Bake for 20 minutes, or until the bottoms are golden brown and the tops are lightly golden.

Per Serving (1 scone of 8): Calories: 277; Fat: 12g; Carbohydrates: 34g; Fiber: 3g; Sugar: 1g; Protein: 7g; Sodium: 456mg

Tomato and Almond Ricotta Toasts

SERVES 4   PREP TIME: 20 MINUTES
ONE-POT, OIL-FREE, SOY-FREE

I love using almond ricotta as an alternative to store-bought vegan cream cheese or as a replacement for hummus or mayonnaise on a sandwich. This version is creamy, tangy, and so easy to make, you'll want to keep it on hand. Luckily, it will last up to a week in the refrigerator. Because you're using almond slivers, you don't have to worry about soaking the nuts overnight. You will still need to use a food processor or high-speed blender, though. Try flavoring your ricotta by stirring in fresh chopped herbs such as oregano, basil, or parsley after you've blended it.

2 cups slivered blanched almonds

3 tablespoons nutritional yeast

2 tablespoons lemon juice

1 teaspoon kosher salt, divided

¼ teaspoon garlic powder

¾ to 1 cup water

8 slices whole-grain or artisan seed bread, toasted

3 large heirloom tomatoes, sliced ¼-inch thick

¼ teaspoon crushed red pepper flakes

½ teaspoon freshly ground black pepper

1. In a food processor fitted with the S blade or in a high-speed blender, combine the almonds, nutritional yeast, lemon juice, ½ teaspoon of salt, the garlic powder, and ¾ cup of water. Process until the mixture is mostly smooth, stopping to scrape down the sides as needed, until only a little bit of almond is visible. If the mixture is too thick to continue blending, add the remaining water, 1 tablespoon at a time, until the right consistency is reached.

2. Layer about ¼ cup of the ricotta on each slice of toast, then add 2 or 3 tomato slices to each and sprinkle with red pepper flakes, black pepper, and the remaining ½ teaspoon of salt before serving.

Cooking Tip: This recipe will create a slightly wetter ricotta. If you'd like it to be firmer and drier, place it in some cheesecloth or a kitchen towel, roll it up to form a ball, and place it in a fine-mesh strainer over a bowl in the refrigerator for a day to firm up.

Per Serving: Calories: 602; Fat: 32g; Carbohydrates: 64g; Fiber: 20g; Sugar: 16g; Protein: 26g; Sodium: 959mg

Tempeh Hash-Stuffed Portobellos

SERVES 4 **PREP TIME:** 10 MINUTES **COOK TIME:** 20 MINUTES
GLUTEN-FREE, NUT-FREE, SOY-FREE

I'm a sucker for any dish that has an edible bowl. It just makes it more fun to eat. Here, the portobello mushroom cap acts as a cradle for delicious potato and pepper hash. What makes this dish successful is the use of frozen hash browns. Choose small, diced potatoes that will cook quickly. I like to use Ore-Ida or Cavendish.

4 portobello mushrooms, stemmed and
    gills removed

¾ teaspoon kosher salt, divided

¾ teaspoon freshly ground black
    pepper, divided

2 tablespoons grapeseed oil

½ cup diced yellow onion

½ cup diced red bell pepper

½ cup diced green bell pepper

1¼ cups diced frozen hash brown potatoes

3 ounces (about 5 strips) tempeh, diced

½ teaspoon chili powder

1. Preheat the oven to 400°F. Line a standard rimmed baking sheet with parchment paper or silicone.

2. Place the mushroom caps on the baking sheet, gill-side up. Sprinkle each mushroom with ⅛ teaspoon of salt and ⅛ teaspoon of black pepper. While your oven is still preheating, bake the mushrooms for 20 minutes.

3. Meanwhile, in a large, deep skillet or cast-iron skillet, heat the oil over medium-high heat until it shimmers. Add the onion, bell peppers, hash browns, tempeh, chili powder, and remaining ¼ teaspoon each of salt and pepper. Toss all the ingredients to combine and cook for 10 to 15 minutes, or until the potatoes are soft and the onions are golden.

4. Remove the mushroom caps from the oven and place them on plates. Scoop the hash into each mushroom and serve.

Cooking Tip: Frozen diced bell peppers and onions are a real time-saver, especially in the morning. Most grocery stores sell these, but if you can't find them, dice up a couple of onions and bell peppers and stash them in freezer-safe bags in your freezer for later use.

Per Serving: Calories: 195; Fat: 10g; Carbohydrates: 22g; Fiber: 4g; Sugar: 5g; Protein: 8g; Sodium: 246mg

Creamy Spinach and Mushroom Oatmeal

SERVES 2 **PREP TIME:** 5 MINUTES **COOK TIME:** 15 MINUTES
ONE-POT, NUT-FREE, OIL-FREE, SOY-FREE

If you're scratching your head at this recipe, you're not alone. I was pretty skeptical the first time I tried making savory oatmeal. To me, it's always been a sweet breakfast dish. But as a girl who generally prefers savory (or salty) over sweet, I had to give this a try. Guess what? It's full of umami flavor. Once you try it, I guarantee it will become your new favorite, too.

2 tablespoons plus 1½ cups no-salt-added
    vegetable broth
1½ cups (6 ounces) sliced cremini
    mushrooms
3 cups packed baby spinach
1 teaspoon jarred minced garlic or 2 garlic
    cloves, minced

1 teaspoon low-sodium tamari
1 cup quick-cooking steel cut oats
¼ cup nutritional yeast
¼ teaspoon kosher salt
¼ teaspoon freshly ground black pepper

1. In a medium pot, heat the 2 tablespoons of broth over medium heat. Add the mushrooms and cook, stirring occasionally, until soft, about 5 minutes. Add the spinach and cook, stirring constantly, until it has wilted, about 3 minutes. Add the garlic and stir for 30 seconds.

2. Pour in the remaining 1½ cups of broth and the tamari, then add the oats. Stir to combine and bring to a boil. Immediately reduce the heat to medium and cook, stirring constantly, until it's as thick as you like it (5 minutes will get it to a thick and creamy consistency without being too stiff).

3. Remove from the heat and stir in the nutritional yeast, salt, and pepper. Serve warm.

Cooking Tip: Mornings can be busy enough without having to do a ton of cooking prep. Choose presliced mushrooms and bagged baby spinach to make this a quick morning meal.

Per Serving: Calories: 397; Fat: 7g; Carbohydrates: 65g; Fiber: 14g; Sugar: 3g; Protein: 24g; Sodium: 460mg

Loaded Breakfast Sweet Potatoes

SERVES 4 **PREP TIME:** 10 MINUTES **COOK TIME:** 20 MINUTES

ONE-POT, GLUTEN-FREE, NUT-FREE, OIL-FREE, SOY-FREE

Sweet potatoes are an excellent breakfast food. Aside from the fact that they are a complex carbohydrate that's high in fiber, vitamins, and minerals, they are hearty and delicious and pair really well with typical breakfast flavors like cinnamon, maple, and nut butters. Sweet potatoes cook quickly in the microwave, too, making this an easy morning meal, even on busy days.

4 medium sweet potatoes, scrubbed

4 tablespoons tahini, divided

2 bananas, sliced

½ cup chopped pitted dates, divided

¼ cup unsweetened shredded coconut, divided

4 tablespoons pure maple syrup, divided

2 tablespoons chia seeds, divided

1. Pierce each sweet potato several times with a fork. Place them on a microwave-safe plate. Microwave for 16 to 20 minutes, or until the potatoes are tender.

2. Remove the potatoes from the microwave and cut lengthwise down the middle of each, about two-thirds of the way through. Use a fork to lightly mash the potato inside.

3. Top each potato with 1 tablespoon of tahini, 5 or 6 banana slices, 2 tablespoons of dates, 1 tablespoon of shredded coconut, 1 tablespoon of maple syrup, and ½ tablespoon of chia seeds. Serve.

Variation Tip: Sweet potatoes are a great canvas for lots of different toppings. Try adding nut butters like peanut, almond, or even cashew, along with cinnamon, nutmeg, chopped dried fruits, and seeds.

Per Serving: Calories: 420; Fat: 13g; Carbohydrates: 74g; Fiber: 12g; Sugar: 37g; Protein: 7g; Sodium: 94mg

Mixed Berry Breakfast Bread Pudding

SERVES 3   PREP TIME: 10 MINUTES   COOK TIME: 15 MINUTES
ONE-POT, OIL-FREE, SOY-FREE

This is truly one of the most comforting breakfast dishes you'll ever make. It tastes like a cross between maple-cinnamon oatmeal and French toast, but with less work. It's also a fantastic way to use up day-old or slightly stale bread, which is always hanging around my house. If you don't have any day-old bread, just lightly toast your bread before using to help dry it out.

6 slices whole-wheat bread, cut or torn into chunks

1½ cups unsweetened vanilla almond milk

1 teaspoon ground cinnamon

¼ teaspoon ground nutmeg

4 cups mixed raspberries, blueberries, blackberries, fresh or frozen

3 tablespoons pure maple syrup

3 teaspoons blueberry jam

1 teaspoon light brown sugar

1. Place the bread chunks in a large skillet. Add the milk and sprinkle the cinnamon and nutmeg over the top.

2. Heat over medium heat to warm (but not boil) the milk, about 5 minutes, or until steaming.

3. Add the mixed berries, maple syrup, and jam and continue to cook for 10 minutes, stirring frequently, or until the bread has absorbed most of the milk.

4. Sprinkle with brown sugar and serve.

Variation Tip: Any soft fruit would work well in this dish, so try swapping the mixed berries and jam for bananas and peanut butter, or blackberries and peaches and apricot jam.

Per Serving: Calories: 402; Fat: 4g; Carbohydrates: 80g; Fiber: 10g; Sugar: 36g; Protein: 13g; Sodium: 502mg

Blueberry Lemon Pancakes

SERVES 2 **PREP TIME:** 10 MINUTES **COOK TIME:** 20 MINUTES
NUT-FREE

These are hands-down the fluffiest vegan pancakes you'll ever have, and I guarantee they will become your weekend favorite. I use baking powder as the egg replacer to give the pancakes a light, fluffy texture, and top with blueberry lemon compote to elevate them into brunch-worthy pancakes. If blueberry isn't your favorite, try swapping it for strawberry or cherry.

FOR THE COMPOTE

2 cups fresh blueberries, divided
2 tablespoons granulated sugar
1 teaspoon lemon zest
2 teaspoons lemon juice
¼ teaspoon kosher salt

FOR THE PANCAKES

1 cup all-purpose flour
1 tablespoon baking powder
2 tablespoons coconut sugar
½ teaspoon kosher salt
½ teaspoon ground cinnamon
2 tablespoons canola oil
1 cup plain unsweetened soy milk
1 teaspoon pure vanilla extract

1. In a medium saucepan, combine 1 cup of blueberries, the granulated sugar, lemon zest, lemon juice, and salt. Heat over medium heat, stirring occasionally, until the blueberries are bubbling and start to break down, about 7 minutes. Remove from the heat and stir in the remaining 1 cup of blueberries. Set aside.

2. Meanwhile, preheat a wide nonstick skillet or griddle pan over low heat. In a large bowl, combine the flour, baking powder, coconut sugar, salt, and cinnamon. Make a well in the center of the bowl and add the oil, soy milk, and vanilla. Whisk to form a batter.

3. Using a ¼-cup measure, scoop a level cupful of batter onto the preheated skillet and smooth it out to form an even circle. Repeat so that you have two pancakes in the skillet. Cook until bubbles and craters form, about 4 minutes, then flip and cook for an additional 2 minutes. Transfer to a plate and repeat with the remaining batter. You should end up with six pancakes. Serve topped with the blueberry compote.

Per Serving (3 pancakes): Calories: 574; Fat: 17g; Carbohydrates: 98g; Fiber: 7g; Sugar: 40g; Protein: 11g; Sodium: 1,463mg

Chocolate Orange French Toast

SERVES 4 **PREP TIME:** 10 MINUTES **COOK TIME:** 20 MINUTES
SOY-FREE

Chocolate and orange is a classic combination. It always makes me think of the holidays, so I tend to save this dish for Sunday mornings in December—but really, it's delicious any time of year. To elevate this French toast to almost dessert status, sprinkle chocolate chips on top and dust it with powdered sugar before serving.

1 tablespoon ground flaxseed

3 tablespoons hot water

2 cups plain unsweetened almond milk

3 tablespoons unsweetened cocoa powder

½ teaspoon ground cinnamon

¼ teaspoon ground nutmeg

2 tablespoons coconut sugar

3 tablespoons orange zest

2 tablespoons orange juice

8 tablespoons vegan butter, divided

8 slices whole-grain bread

1. Make a flax egg by combining the flaxseed with the hot water in a small bowl. Stir and let it sit for 2 to 3 minutes until thickened.

2. In a shallow dish, combine the flax egg, almond milk, cocoa powder, cinnamon, nutmeg, sugar, orange zest, and orange juice. Set aside.

3. In a large nonstick skillet, melt 2 tablespoons of vegan butter over medium heat.

4. Dip a slice of bread into the almond milk mixture for 3 to 5 seconds. Remove and let the excess milk drip back into the bowl. Repeat with a second slice.

5. Place the 2 slices of bread into the skillet with the melted butter and cook for 3 to 4 minutes per side. Transfer to a plate. Repeat with the remaining bread slices and serve.

Per Serving (2 slices): Calories: 486; Fat: 27g; Carbohydrates: 50g; Fiber: 8g; Sugar: 12g; Protein: 13g; Sodium: 699mg

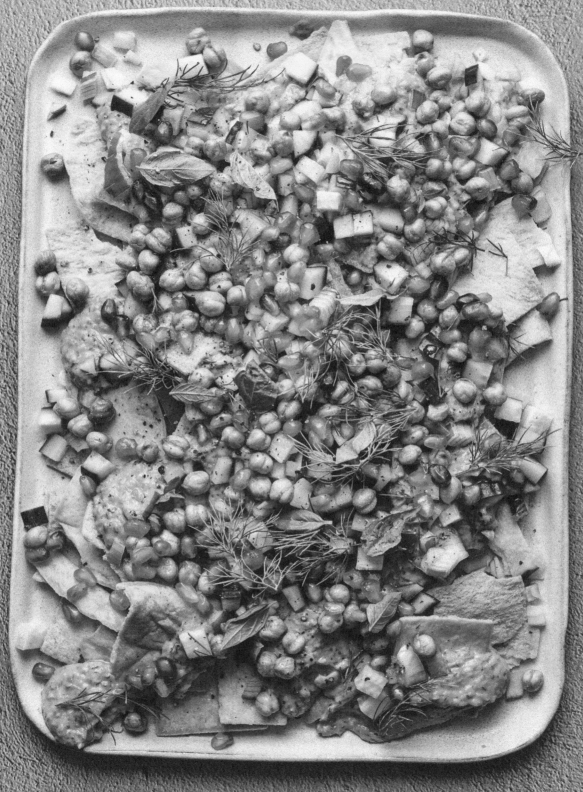

GREEN GODDESS DIP NACHOS, P.40

3

Snacks & Bites

Sweet Chili Edamame   30

Chipotle Peanut Sesame Salsa   31

Spicy Tahini Cauliflower Wings   32

Sun-Dried Tomato and
White Bean Hummus Flatbreads   33

Smoked "Salmon" Crostini   34

Raspberry PB&J Muffins   36

Baked Chickpea "Chick'n" Nuggets   37

Pepperoncini and Roasted Red Pepper
Garlic Bread Pinwheels   38

Moo Shu Lettuce Cups   39

Green Goddess Dip Nachos   40

Sweet Chili Edamame

SERVES 3   **PREP TIME:** 5 MINUTES   **COOK TIME:** 5 MINUTES
ONE-POT, GLUTEN-FREE, NUT-FREE

In my house, we Netflix and snack, so I'm always looking for healthier munchies to indulge in. It's easy to rip open a bag of potato chips, but all that processing, frying, and salt isn't healthy—and we never feel great afterward. Luckily, I always have precooked frozen edamame in my freezer and my kids will happily eat them anytime. To make this snack super quick, I cook my edamame in the microwave while I assemble the sauce on the stove.

3 cups frozen edamame pods

3 tablespoons Thai sweet chili sauce

½ teaspoon jarred minced garlic or 1 garlic clove, minced

1 teaspoon sesame oil

¼ teaspoon kosher salt

2 teaspoons sesame seeds

1.   In a medium microwave-safe bowl, microwave the edamame according to the package directions.

2.   Meanwhile, whisk together the Thai chili sauce, garlic, oil, salt, and sesame seeds in a small pot. Heat over medium heat until just warmed through, about 3 minutes.

3.   Toss the edamame with the sauce until coated and serve.

Per Serving: Calories: 186; Fat: 9g; Carbohydrates: 19g; Fiber: 6g; Sugar: 12g; Protein: 14g; Sodium: 369mg

Chipotle Peanut Sesame Salsa

MAKES 3 CUPS   PREP TIME: 10 MINUTES
GLUTEN-FREE, OIL-FREE, SOY-FREE

Shake up your snack game with this nutty, spicy twist on classic nachos and salsa. This version combines smoky and sweet flavors in a creamy peanut salsa with just enough heat to tickle your taste buds. You can make this salsa nut-free by swapping peanut butter for an equal amount of well-stirred tahini. Tahini has a naturally nutty flavor but is made entirely from sesame seeds. I like to serve this salsa with a mix of red, yellow, and blue corn chips, but it also makes a fabulous dip for veggies.

1 (15-ounce) can diced tomatoes, drained

½ medium yellow onion, diced

1 teaspoon jarred minced garlic or 2 garlic cloves, minced

½ cup creamy unsalted peanut butter

1 large chipotle pepper in adobo sauce

2 tablespoons fresh lime juice

1 cup chopped fresh cilantro or flat-leaf parsley

½ teaspoon ground cumin

½ teaspoon kosher salt

1.   Combine the tomatoes, onion, garlic, peanut butter, chipotle pepper, lime juice, cilantro, cumin, and salt in a food processor or blender and pulse until smooth.

2.   Transfer to a bowl and enjoy immediately.

Ingredient Tip: Chipotle in adobo is a great way to add smoky hot flavor to a dish. Chipotle in adobo sauce is smoked, dried, and rehydrated jalapeño peppers that are packed in a tangy pureed sauce made from tomatoes, garlic, vinegar, and spices. It has become so popular that you can easily find it in the Mexican foods section of your supermarket.

Per Serving (¼ cup): Calories: 77; Fat: 5g; Carbohydrates: 5g; Fiber: 2g; Sugar: 2g; Protein: 3g; Sodium: 169mg

Spicy Tahini Cauliflower Wings

SERVES 4   **PREP TIME:** 5 MINUTES   **COOK TIME:** 20 MINUTES
GLUTEN-FREE, NUT-FREE, OIL-FREE, SOY-FREE

This is a fantastic snack or appetizer that goes beyond the standard plate of cauliflower wings. Tahini and rice vinegar add a sharp, nutty flavor that blends so well with the cumin and chili. I like serving this dish on a bed of deep green lettuce or kale leaves, which contrasts nicely with the bright golden hue of these baked cauliflower bites. To keep prep time to a minimum, use bagged precut fresh cauliflower florets.

1 (500g) bag fresh precut cauliflower florets

¼ cup rice vinegar

2 tablespoons tahini

2 teaspoons pure maple syrup

1 teaspoon ground cumin

½ teaspoon ground turmeric

½ teaspoon kosher salt

¼ teaspoon crushed red pepper flakes, plus more as needed

1. Preheat the oven to 400°F and line a large baking sheet with parchment paper.

2. Spread the cauliflower florets on the baking sheet in an even, single layer and set aside.

3. In a small bowl, whisk together the rice vinegar, tahini, maple syrup, cumin, turmeric, salt, and red pepper flakes until well combined. Pour over the cauliflower florets and use your hands to toss them until well coated.

4. Bake for 15 to 20 minutes, or until golden. Serve immediately.

Per Serving: Calories: 88; Fat: 4g; Carbohydrates: 10g; Fiber: 4g; Sugar: 5g; Protein: 4g; Sodium: 342mg

Sun-Dried Tomato and White Bean Hummus Flatbreads

SERVES 6   **PREP TIME:** 20 MINUTES   **COOK TIME:** 5 MINUTES
NUT-FREE, OIL-FREE, SOY-FREE

This warm white bean hummus is a great alternative to traditional hummus and makes a great hot snack when served on lightly toasted naan or other flatbreads. I use oil-packed tomatoes to avoid additional oil while cooking. If you don't have oil-packed, use regular ones and add a teaspoon or two of oil to your skillet before cooking.

3 pieces vegan naan

2 (14-ounce cans) no-salt-added cannellini beans, drained and rinsed

½ cup no-salt-added vegetable broth

6 jarred sun-dried tomatoes, chopped and lightly patted dry

1 teaspoon jarred minced garlic or 2 garlic cloves, minced

2 tablespoons lemon juice

¼ cup nutritional yeast

¼ teaspoon kosher salt

¼ teaspoon freshly ground black pepper

3 tablespoons minced fresh parsley (optional)

1. Preheat the oven to 425°F. Line a baking sheet with parchment paper.

2. Place the naan on the lined baking sheet and warm in the oven for 4 to 5 minutes while you make the white bean spread.

3. In a food processor fitted with the S blade, combine the beans and vegetable broth and pulse until coarsely chopped. (You could also do this in a large bowl with a potato masher or a fork.) Set aside.

4. In a large skillet, heat the sun-dried tomatoes and garlic over medium-high heat. Cook for 2 to 3 minutes, or until fragrant. Add the mashed white bean mixture and cook, stirring frequently, until warmed through, about 5 minutes. Remove from the heat and stir in the lemon juice, nutritional yeast, salt, and pepper.

5. Spread the mix evenly over the naan and sprinkle with parsley (if using). Quarter each piece of naan and serve.

Per Serving (2 pieces): Calories: 256; Fat: 4g; Carbohydrates: 42g; Fiber: 9g; Sugar: 2g; Protein: 14g; Sodium: 286mg

Smoked "Salmon" Crostini

SERVES 8 **PREP TIME:** 15 MINUTES **COOK TIME:** 10 MINUTES
NUT-FREE, OIL-FREE

Smoked salmon spread is a classic snack (and great on a bagel, too!). I've created a fishless version by using brined vegetables to mimic the salty flavor of smoked salmon and simulated bacon bits to add smokiness. This recipe uses store-bought vegan cream cheese (I prefer Daiya or Tofutti plain vegan cream cheese for this recipe) and processed bacon bits, but if you prefer not to use these kinds of products, swap them for an equal amount of medium tofu and a couple of drops of liquid smoke.

1 large French baguette, cut on the bias into
 1-inch-thick slices

6 jarred sun-dried tomatoes, patted dry

12 pitted kalamata olives, finely chopped

2 tablespoons drained and chopped capers

¼ cup drained and chopped roasted
 red peppers

2 tablespoons prepared horseradish

¼ cup simulated bacon bits

2 tablespoons coconut sugar

½ teaspoon kosher salt

2 (8-ounce) containers plain vegan cream
 cheese, at room temperature

1 tablespoon lemon juice

Dill sprigs, for garnish (optional)

6 lemon wedges (optional)

1. Preheat the oven to 400°F.

2. Arrange the baguette slices on a rimmed baking sheet and place them in the oven while it's still preheating. Toast for 5 to 7 minutes so that they crisp up but aren't dark.

3. Meanwhile, make the spread. In a large bowl, mix together the sun-dried tomatoes, olives, capers, roasted red peppers, horseradish, bacon bits, sugar, and salt. Add the cream cheese and lemon juice and mix until well combined.

4. Remove the baguette toasts from the oven and spread about 1½ tablespoons of the spread on each one. Arrange on a serving platter, placing any leftover dip in a small ramekin to serve on the side.

5. If using, garnish with dill and lemon wedges, and enjoy.

Ingredient Tip: Did you know that most brands of simulated bacon bits are actually both vegan and gluten-free? They are a fantastic addition to vegan dips, salads, and soups.

Per Serving (1 of 8): Calories: 286; Fat: 17g; Carbohydrates: 30g; Fiber: 2g; Sugar: 4g; Protein: 5g; Sodium: 823mg

Raspberry PB&J Muffins

MAKES 12 MUFFINS **PREP TIME:** 10 MINUTES **COOK TIME:** 20 MINUTES
OIL-FREE, SOY-FREE

We all know that muffins are a great on-the-go snack, and we also know there's nothing more comforting than a classic PB&J sandwich. So why not combine the two? Whole-wheat flour gives these muffins extra protein and fiber, and just a touch of brown sugar adds a caramelized, nutty flavor. I love raspberries and raspberry jam, but if you're partial to a classic strawberry-jam PB&J, go right ahead and swap it in.

1½ cups whole-wheat flour

¼ cup packed light brown sugar

2 teaspoons baking powder

½ teaspoon kosher salt

½ cup creamy unsalted peanut butter

½ cup unsweetened applesauce

1 cup plain unsweetened almond milk

½ cup all-natural raspberry jam (seedless if possible), divided

½ pint fresh raspberries

1. Preheat the oven to 375°F. Line a 12-cup muffin tin with paper liners and set aside.

2. In a large bowl, whisk together the flour, brown sugar, baking powder, and salt. Add the peanut butter and, using either a pastry cutter or two knives working in a crisscross motion, cut the peanut butter into the dry ingredients until it resembles coarse crumbs. Add the applesauce and milk and stir until a lumpy batter forms.

3. Fill each muffin cup one-quarter full of the batter, then add ½ teaspoon of raspberry jam to each one and top with the remaining batter, filling each cup no more than three-quarters full.

4. Top each muffin with 2 to 3 raspberries. Bake for 15 to 18 minutes, or until a toothpick inserted in the center comes out with only jam on it. Enjoy.

Per Serving (1 muffin): Calories: 166; Fat: 6g; Carbohydrates: 26g; Fiber: 3g; Sugar: 12g; Protein: 5g; Sodium: 203mg

Baked Chickpea "Chick'n" Nuggets

SERVES 2 **PREP TIME:** 15 MINUTES **COOK TIME:** 15 MINUTES
FREEZER-FRIENDLY, GLUTEN-FREE, OIL-FREE, SOY-FREE

I have small kids, which means chick'n nuggets are a staple in my house. And while it is convenient to keep a bag of store-bought vegan nuggets in the freezer, it's not the healthiest option. That's why I love these nuggets. They take the same amount of time to make as the frozen kind but use whole ingredients and are free from soy and gluten. Most important, my kids love them. They freeze well, too, so consider making a larger batch and storing them in a freezer-safe bag for up to 3 months.

2 (15-ounce) cans no-salt-added chickpeas, drained and rinsed

1 medium yellow onion, roughly chopped

½ cup gluten-free oats

1 teaspoon yellow mustard

1 tablespoon nutritional yeast

1 teaspoon onion powder

1 teaspoon garlic powder

½ teaspoon smoked paprika

½ teaspoon kosher salt

½ cup plain unsweetened almond milk

¾ cup crushed vegan cornflakes

1. Preheat the oven to 350°F. Line a standard baking sheet with parchment paper.

2. In a food processor fitted with an S blade or a high-speed blender, combine the chickpeas, onion, oats, mustard, nutritional yeast, onion and garlic powders, smoked paprika, and salt and pulse until smooth.

3. Create a breading station by placing the almond milk and cornflakes in two small bowls. Scoop 2 heaping tablespoons of the chickpea mixture into your hands and form it into a nugget shape. Dip it into the almond milk and then the cornflakes.

4. Place on the prepared baking sheet and repeat with all of the remaining mix. Bake for 15 minutes, or until lightly golden.

Variation Tip: This recipe can either be nut-free or soy-free depending on which plant-based milk you choose. If you go with gluten-free oat milk, it's both! Also, if you can't find vegan cornflakes, you can swap them out for panko bread crumbs.

Per Serving: Calories: 545; Fat: 10g; Carbohydrates: 92g; Fiber: 22g; Sugar: 15g; Protein: 26g; Sodium: 995mg

Pepperoncini and Roasted Red Pepper Garlic Bread Pinwheels

SERVES 4 PREP TIME: 10 MINUTES **COOK TIME:** 15 MINUTES
NUT-FREE, SOY-FREE

While I was growing up, my dad was the king of garlic bread, and it was a given that if the big game was on TV or it was card night, a platter of garlic bread would be included. In this version, mildly spicy pickled pepperoncini peppers add a punch of flavor and pair well with juicy roasted red peppers. It's the perfect way to jazz up garlic bread.

6 tablespoons vegan butter, softened

2 teaspoons jarred minced garlic or 4 garlic cloves, minced

1 tablespoon chopped fresh flat-leaf parsley or 1½ teaspoons dried parsley

1 loaf French or Italian bread

¼ cup jarred roasted red peppers, patted dry and finely chopped

¼ cup chopped pepperoncini peppers

1 cup marinara sauce (optional)

1. Preheat the oven to 375°F. Line a standard baking tray with parchment paper or foil.

2. In a small bowl, combine the butter, garlic, and parsley and mix well.

3. Halve the bread lengthwise and spread the garlic butter evenly over both halves. Top with the roasted red peppers and pepperoncini peppers. Bake for 10 to 12 minutes, or until the edges are golden.

4. Cut into slices and serve with marinara sauce for dipping (if using).

Ingredient Tip: Roasted red peppers are a powerhouse of smoky sweet flavor that can brighten up any dish. Use the leftover peppers from the jar to make a roasted red pepper sauce for pasta, or mix with cream cheese for a savory breakfast treat. They are also a great addition to Easy Lahmajoun (page 64) or as a replacement for the sun-dried tomatoes in Sun-Dried Tomato and Zucchini Scones (page 20).

Per Serving: Calories: 459; Fat: 18g; Carbohydrates: 61g; Fiber: 2g; Sugar: 1g; Protein: 10g; Sodium: 988mg

Moo Shu Lettuce Cups

SERVES 6 **PREP TIME:** 15 MINUTES **COOK TIME:** 12 MINUTES
ONE-POT, GLUTEN-FREE, NUT-FREE

These lettuce cups are so full of deep, earthy umami flavor that even the most hardcore omnivore won't notice they are meat-free. Cremini mushrooms and hoisin sauce provide a deep, meaty flavor while water chestnuts add great texture and crunch.

2 tablespoons sesame oil

5 scallions, finely chopped

6 large cremini mushrooms, stemmed and caps diced

¼ cup canned water chestnuts, drained and diced

2 teaspoons jarred minced ginger

1 teaspoon jarred minced garlic or 2 garlic cloves, minced

1 (14-ounce) bag coleslaw mix

1 tablespoon rice wine or red wine vinegar

1 tablespoon low-sodium tamari

2 tablespoons gluten-free hoisin sauce, plus more for topping

1 head Bibb, Boston, or iceberg lettuce, bottom core cut out and leaves separated to use as cups

1. In a large skillet, heat the oil over medium-high heat until it shimmers. Add the scallions, mushrooms, water chestnuts, ginger, and garlic and cook until the mushrooms start to brown, about 4 minutes.

2. Add the coleslaw mix and cook, stirring constantly, for 5 minutes. Add the vinegar, tamari, and hoisin sauce and continue cooking, tossing to coat, for 2 minutes.

3. Remove from the heat and serve immediately with lettuce cups.

Ingredient Tip: Water chestnuts are typically canned and packed in water. You can find them in the Asian foods section of most grocery stores. Choose sliced instead of whole to shorten your prep time.

Per Serving: Calories: 87; Fat: 5g; Carbohydrates: 10g; Fiber: 3g; Sugar: 5g; Protein: 3g; Sodium: 224mg

Green Goddess Dip Nachos

SERVES 5 **PREP TIME:** 30 MINUTES
ONE-POT, NUT-FREE, SOY-FREE

This is a really fun way to shake up a plate of nachos. I've swapped traditional tortilla chips for baked pita chips (I like Stacy's) and turned a fresh, herbal green goddess dressing into the perfect dip. I've paired it with fresh, crisp cucumber, sharp red onion, and roasted chickpeas to add flavor and texture. Since typical green goddess dip includes feta cheese, you could add your favorite store-bought vegan feta as an additional topping.

FOR THE GREEN GODDESS DIP

1 (15-ounce) can no-salt-added white beans, drained and rinsed

1 teaspoon jarred minced garlic or 2 garlic cloves, minced

1 large avocado, peeled and pitted

Juice of 1 lemon

½ cup roughly chopped fresh dill

½ cup roughly chopped fresh basil

½ cup roughly chopped scallions

1 teaspoon Dijon mustard

1 tablespoon extra-virgin olive oil

¼ cup water, plus more as needed

½ teaspoon kosher salt

½ teaspoon freshly ground black pepper

FOR THE NACHO PLATTER

1 (18-ounce) bag toasted pita chips

½ seedless cucumber, diced

½ red onion, diced

¾ cup roasted chickpeas, homemade (see tip) or store-bought

1 cup pomegranate seeds

1. In a blender or food processor, combine the beans, garlic, avocado, lemon juice, dill, basil, scallions, mustard, oil, water, salt, and pepper. Pulse until smooth. Check the consistency and add additional water if needed. It should be scoopable but still slightly pourable.

2. Spread the pita chips on a platter in an even layer.

3. Pour or scoop the dip over the pita chips. Top with cucumber and red onion, then sprinkle with roasted chickpeas and pomegranate seeds before serving.

Cooking Tip: To make your own roasted chickpeas, preheat the oven to 425°F and line a rimmed baking sheet with parchment paper. Drain and rinse 1 (15-ounce) can of no-salt-added chickpeas and place them on the prepared baking sheet. Drizzle with olive oil, salt, and pepper and roast for 20 to 25 minutes, or until golden.

Per Serving: Calories: 772; Fat: 29g; Carbohydrates: 112g; Fiber: 20g; Sugar: 13g; Protein: 20g; Sodium: 1,297mg

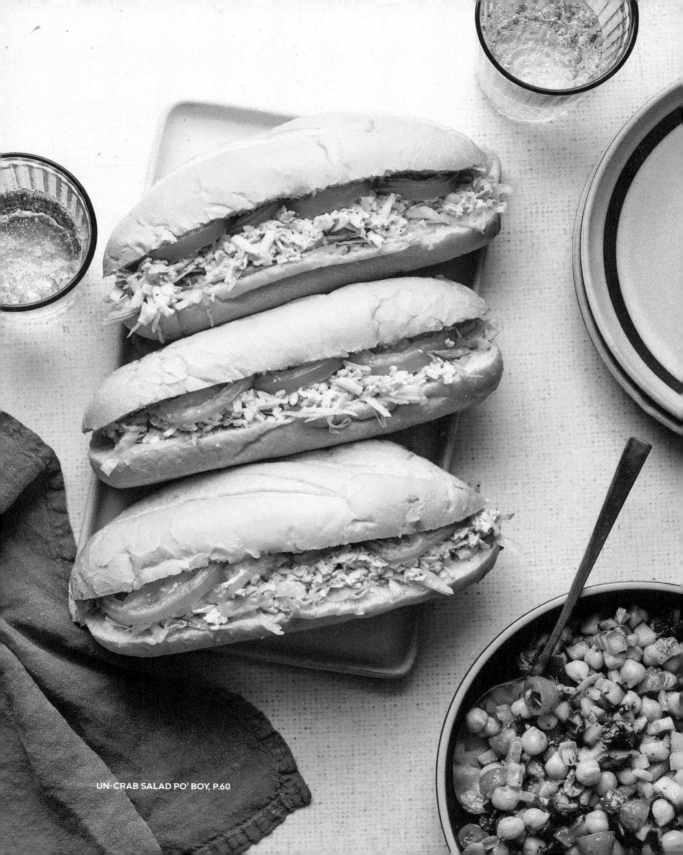

UN-CRAB SALAD PO' BOY, P.60

4

Soups, Salads & Sandwiches

Golden Gazpacho   44

Pumpkin Coconut Soup   45

Tortilla Soup   46

Mediterranean-Inspired Red Lentil Soup   47

Speedy Potato Corn Chowder   48

Lemon Quinoa Artichoke Salad   49

Chili Tofu, Avocado, and Black Bean Salad   50

Mixed Bean and Corn Salad   51

Middle Eastern–Inspired Chopped Chickpea Salad   52

Fiery Curry Pasta Salad   53

Not-Tuna Melt   54

Buffalo Smashed Chickpea Sandwich   56

Jerk Jackfruit Wraps   57

Nashville Hot Tofu Sandwich   58

Un-Crab Salad Po' Boy   60

Golden Gazpacho

SERVES 4 **PREP TIME:** 30 MINUTES
ONE-POT, FREEZER-FRIENDLY, GLUTEN-FREE, NUT-FREE, SOY-FREE

Gazpacho is a wonderfully refreshing cold soup that is perfect on hot summer days. This golden gazpacho incorporates the bright, bold flavors of curry powder and turmeric with less-acidic yellow tomatoes for a soup that is velvety smooth and full of flavor. Gazpacho lasts for up to 5 days in the refrigerator or up to 3 months in the freezer, making this a fabulous big-batch dish.

2 pounds yellow tomatoes

1 large yellow bell pepper, seeded and roughly chopped

1 large yellow onion, roughly chopped

1 cucumber, peeled, seeded, and roughly chopped

1 garlic clove, peeled

2 tablespoons extra-virgin olive oil

2 tablespoons white wine vinegar

½ teaspoon mild curry powder

¼ teaspoon ground turmeric

½ teaspoon kosher salt

½ teaspoon freshly ground black pepper

1. In a blender or food processor, combine the tomatoes, bell pepper, onion, cucumber, garlic, oil, and vinegar and process until smooth.

2. Add the curry powder, turmeric, salt, and black pepper and pulse to combine.

3. Strain through a fine-mesh sieve into a large bowl, using a ladle and working in a circular motion. Taste and adjust the seasonings as needed. Serve immediately or chill in the refrigerator.

Ingredient Tip: Two pounds of yellow tomatoes is about 5 medium tomatoes or 3 pints of cherry tomatoes.

Per Serving: Calories: 139; Fat: 8g; Carbohydrates: 17g; Fiber: 5g; Sugar: 10g; Protein: 3g; Sodium: 311mg

Pumpkin Coconut Soup

SERVES 6   PREP TIME: 10 MINUTES   **COOK TIME:** 20 MINUTES
FREEZER-FRIENDLY, GLUTEN-FREE, NUT-FREE, SOY-FREE

This soup is full of the flavors we associate with fall, like pumpkin, cinnamon, and nutmeg. And it gets a little kick from cayenne—which is totally optional if you're not a fan of spicy food. I love serving this for dinner with some toasted garlic baguette slices and a side salad.

1 tablespoon grapeseed oil or extra-virgin olive oil

½ large yellow onion, roughly chopped

2 tablespoons jarred minced ginger

1 teaspoon jarred minced garlic or 2 garlic cloves, minced

1 (16-ounce) carton low-sodium vegetable broth

1 (15-ounce) can plain pumpkin puree

½ teaspoon ground cinnamon

¼ teaspoon ground nutmeg

¼ teaspoon ground cayenne pepper

½ teaspoon kosher salt

½ teaspoon freshly ground black pepper

1 cup canned light coconut milk

1. In a large soup pot, heat the oil over medium-high heat until it shimmers. Add the onion and ginger and cook until the onion is soft, about 5 minutes, stirring frequently. Add the garlic and cook, stirring constantly, for 30 seconds.

2. Add the vegetable broth and pumpkin, then stir in the cinnamon, nutmeg, cayenne pepper, salt, and black pepper. Bring to a boil, then reduce heat to a simmer and cook, covered, for 10 minutes. Stir in the coconut milk.

3. Remove from the heat and puree the soup by using an immersion blender directly in the pot, or transfer to a blender and blend in small batches. Serve immediately.

Per Serving: Calories: 90; Fat: 5g; Carbohydrates: 10g; Fiber: 2g; Sugar: 4g; Protein: 1g; Sodium: 212mg

Tortilla Soup

SERVES 4   **PREP TIME:** 10 MINUTES   **COOK TIME:** 20 MINUTES
ONE-POT, FREEZER-FRIENDLY, GLUTEN-FREE, NUT-FREE, SOY-FREE

Tortilla soup is a tomato-based soup that is full of bright, bold chili flavor.
I like to pack mine full of protein by adding both black beans and kidney beans,
and I use frozen diced veggies to add nutrients without spending a lot of time doing
prep. I chose butternut squash for this version, but you can use any fresh or frozen
vegetables. In fact, I love to make this soup when I've got to clean out the refrigerator or freezer, because it's a perfect canvas for any quick-cooking veggies.

FOR THE SOUP

1 tablespoon grapeseed oil or extra-virgin
   olive oil

1 medium yellow onion, diced

2 teaspoons jarred minced garlic or 4 garlic
   cloves, minced

1 (28-ounce) can diced tomatoes

3 cups low-sodium vegetable broth

1 tablespoon chili powder

1 teaspoon dried oregano

2 cups frozen diced butternut squash

1 (14-ounce) can no-salt-added black beans,
   drained and rinsed

1 (14-ounce) can no-salt-added red kidney
   beans, drained and rinsed

1 cup frozen corn kernels

OPTIONAL TOPPINGS

1 avocado, cubed

1 lime, quartered

½ cup chopped fresh cilantro

¼ cup dairy-free sour cream

1 cup store-bought tortilla strip
   salad toppers

2 tablespoons pickled jalapeño peppers

1. In a large soup pot, heat the oil over medium-high heat until it shimmers. Add
   the onion and cook, stirring frequently, until just softened, about 4 minutes. Add
   the garlic and cook, stirring constantly, for 30 seconds.

2. Pour in the tomatoes with their juices and the vegetable broth. Add the chili
   powder, oregano, butternut squash, black beans, and kidney beans and bring to a
   boil. Immediately reduce the heat to medium-low and simmer for 10 minutes.

3. Stir in the corn kernels and remove from the heat. (The residual heat will cook
   the corn.) Divide into bowls and add any toppings you'd like.

Per Serving: Calories: 383; Fat: 6g; Carbohydrates: 70g; Fiber: 21g; Sugar: 14g; Protein: 17g; Sodium: 516mg

Mediterranean-Inspired Red Lentil Soup

SERVES 4 **PREP TIME:** 10 MINUTES **COOK TIME:** 20 MINUTES
ONE-POT, FREEZER-FRIENDLY, GLUTEN-FREE, NUT-FREE, SOY-FREE

It is absolutely possible to make a delicious, hearty lentil soup in under 30 minutes. The trick is using split red lentils, which take less time to cook. For this soup, we're infusing classic Mediterranean flavors like cumin, oregano, lemon, and red pepper flakes to add a bold punch of flavor. I like to puree lentil soup to give it a creamy consistency, but it's not necessary.

2 teaspoons grapeseed oil or extra-virgin olive oil

1 cup frozen diced carrots

1 cup frozen diced onions

1 teaspoon jarred minced garlic or 2 garlic cloves, minced

3 teaspoons dried oregano

1 teaspoon ground cumin

½ teaspoon crushed red pepper flakes

Zest of 2 lemons

1 cup canned no-salt-added crushed tomatoes

7 cups low-sodium vegetable broth

2 cups uncooked split red lentils

½ teaspoon kosher salt

Juice of 2 lemons

1. In a large soup pot, heat the oil over medium-high heat until it shimmers. Add the carrots, onions, garlic, oregano, cumin, red pepper flakes, and lemon zest and cook, stirring constantly, until the onions and carrots start to soften, about 4 minutes.

2. Add the crushed tomatoes with their juices, vegetable broth, lentils, and salt and bring to a boil. Immediately reduce the heat to a simmer, cover, and cook for 15 to 20 minutes, or until the lentils are fully cooked.

3. Remove from the heat and puree slightly with an immersion blender to give the soup a creamy consistency, or transfer in small batches to a blender, blend, and return to the pot. Stir in the lemon juice and serve.

Variation Tip: Give yourself a boost of iron and key vitamins B_2 and K by stirring 2 packed cups of baby spinach into the soup just before serving.

Per Serving: Calories: 475; Fat: 4g; Carbohydrates: 83g; Fiber: 17g; Sugar: 10g; Protein: 29g; Sodium: 404mg

Speedy Potato Corn Chowder

SERVES 8 PREP TIME: 10 MINUTES **COOK TIME:** 20 MINUTES
ONE-POT, FREEZER-FRIENDLY, NUT-FREE

I love making this soup on cold winter nights. It's easy enough for a weeknight meal but tastes like it was slow-simmered all day. To help this dish cook quickly, cut your potatoes into really small pieces so that they take less time to boil.

1 tablespoon grapeseed oil or extra-virgin olive oil

1 medium yellow onion, chopped

8 cups low-sodium vegetable broth

3 large yellow potatoes, peeled and cubed

½ cup plain unsweetened soy milk

⅓ cup all-purpose flour

½ teaspoon kosher salt

½ teaspoon freshly ground black pepper

1 teaspoon powdered mustard

1 teaspoon paprika

¼ teaspoon ground nutmeg

2 cups frozen corn

2 cups frozen peas and carrots

1. In a large soup pot, heat the oil over medium-high heat until it shimmers. Add the onion and cook until just soft, about 4 minutes. Add the vegetable broth and potatoes and bring to a boil, then reduce the heat to a simmer and cook until the potatoes are tender, 10 to 15 minutes.

2. Meanwhile, in a small bowl, combine the soy milk, flour, salt, pepper, mustard, paprika, and nutmeg.

3. When the potatoes are tender, stir in the milk mixture along with the frozen corn, peas, and carrots. Bring to a boil and cook, stirring constantly, for 2 to 3 minutes, or until the soup has thickened. Serve.

Per Serving: Calories: 170; Fat: 3g; Carbohydrates: 34g; Fiber: 5g; Sugar: 6g; Protein: 6g; Sodium: 244mg

Lemon Quinoa Artichoke Salad

SERVES 4 **PREP TIME:** 10 MINUTES **COOK TIME:** 20 MINUTES
GLUTEN-FREE, NUT-FREE, SOY-FREE

This is a wonderfully fresh salad that is perfect served warm or chilled. The combination of artichokes, olives, lemon, and olive oil give it a bright Mediterranean vibe. You can easily customize this salad to include whatever vegetables you have on hand, such as arugula, baby spinach, bell peppers, or even diced seedless cucumbers.

2 cups water

1 cup quinoa

1 (13-ounce) can artichokes, drained and chopped

¾ cup grape tomatoes, halved

1 (15-ounce) can no-salt-added chickpeas, drained and rinsed

1 (2.5-ounce) can sliced black olives, drained

¼ cup extra-virgin olive oil

¼ cup lemon juice

1 teaspoon jarred minced garlic or 2 garlic cloves, minced

½ teaspoon kosher salt

½ teaspoon freshly ground black pepper

½ cup chopped fresh flat-leaf parsley

1. In a medium saucepan, combine the water and quinoa and bring to a boil. Reduce the heat to medium-low, cover, and cook until the quinoa is soft and all the water is absorbed, 15 to 20 minutes.

2. Meanwhile, in a large bowl, combine the artichokes, tomatoes, chickpeas, and olives. Set aside.

3. In a small bowl, whisk together the oil, lemon juice, garlic, salt, and pepper. Set aside.

4. Add the cooked quinoa to the vegetables, pour in the dressing, and add the parsley. Toss to combine before enjoying.

Per Serving: Calories: 446; Fat: 20g; Carbohydrates: 59g; Fiber: 16g; Sugar: 8g; Protein: 13g; Sodium: 680mg

Chili Tofu, Avocado, and Black Bean Salad

SERVES 4 **PREP TIME:** 15 MINUTES **COOK TIME:** 15 MINUTES
GLUTEN-FREE, NUT-FREE, OIL-FREE

This salad packs a huge punch of Southwestern flavor and is a great addition to any backyard barbecue or summer party. It's hearty enough to eat on its own or to serve over a bed of crisp greens. To cook the tofu quickly, put it in the oven while it's still preheating and include that as part of your overall cook time.

1 (12-ounce) block extra-firm tofu, cubed

2 tablespoons chili powder

2 cups grape tomatoes, halved

1 orange or yellow bell pepper, seeded and diced

2 medium ripe avocados, cubed

2 scallions, diced

1 (15-ounce) can no-salt-added black beans, drained and rinsed

¼ cup lime juice

2 tablespoons white wine vinegar or apple cider vinegar

2 teaspoons agave syrup or pure maple syrup

½ teaspoon kosher salt

½ teaspoon freshly ground black pepper

1. Preheat the oven to 425°F. Line a standard baking sheet with parchment paper.

2. Combine the tofu and chili powder in a large resealable bag and shake well to coat. Spread out the tofu cubes on the prepared baking sheet and bake for 15 minutes.

3. Meanwhile, in a large bowl, combine the tomatoes, bell pepper, avocados, scallions, and beans.

4. In a small bowl, whisk together the lime juice, vinegar, syrup, salt, and black pepper.

5. Add the cooked tofu to the mixed vegetables, pour on the dressing, and toss to coat. Serve immediately.

Per Serving: Calories: 360; Fat: 16g; Carbohydrates: 44g; Fiber: 17g; Sugar: 6g; Protein: 19g; Sodium: 283mg

Mixed Bean and Corn Salad

SERVES 6   PREP TIME: 20 MINUTES
GLUTEN-FREE, NUT-FREE, SOY-FREE

This is a high-fiber, protein-packed salad that is so simple and delicious, you'll want to have it on constant repeat. It makes a hearty lunch on top of greens or in a wrap, and it is a fantastic alternative to starch-heavy rice or potatoes as a side dish.

1 (15-ounce) can no-salt-added red kidney beans, drained and rinsed

1 (15-ounce) can no-salt-added pinto beans, drained and rinsed

1 (15-ounce) can no-salt-added chickpeas, drained and rinsed

1 (8-ounce) can no-salt-added corn, drained

½ medium red onion, diced

¼ cup chopped fresh flat-leaf parsley

⅓ cup extra-virgin olive oil

⅓ cup red wine vinegar

2 tablespoons lemon juice

½ teaspoon dried oregano

½ teaspoon chili powder

½ teaspoon kosher salt

½ teaspoon freshly ground black pepper

1. In a large bowl, combine the kidney beans, pinto beans, chickpeas, corn, red onion, and parsley.

2. In a small bowl, whisk together the oil, vinegar, lemon juice, oregano, chili powder, salt, and pepper. Pour over the mixed beans and toss to coat. Serve.

Per Serving: Calories: 323; Fat: 14g; Carbohydrates: 39g; Fiber: 9g; Sugar: 6g; Protein: 12g; Sodium: 198mg

Middle Eastern–Inspired Chopped Chickpea Salad

SERVES 4 **PREP TIME:** 20 MINUTES
GLUTEN-FREE, NUT-FREE, SOY-FREE

I love the bold spices and bright, fresh flavors of Middle Eastern food. Growing up, we had a favorite falafel restaurant and they made this chopped salad that I could eat by the bucketful. It was used as a condiment or side dish, but I turned it into a full salad by adding protein-packed chickpeas. I like to serve it nestled into a bed of creamy hummus with some fresh pita.

2 (15-ounce) cans no-salt-added chickpeas, drained and rinsed

1 pint (2 cups) grape tomatoes, halved

2 seedless cucumbers, finely chopped

1 small red onion, diced

1 cup chopped pitted kalamata olives

½ cup chopped pitted green olives

1 cup chopped fresh flat-leaf parsley

¼ cup extra-virgin olive oil

¼ cup lemon juice

½ teaspoon ground cumin

½ teaspoon ground sumac

½ teaspoon kosher salt

½ teaspoon freshly ground black pepper

1. In a large bowl, combine the chickpeas, tomatoes, cucumbers, onion, olives, and parsley. Set aside.

2. In a small bowl, whisk together the oil, lemon juice, cumin, sumac, salt, and pepper. Pour over the chopped vegetables and toss to coat before serving.

Ingredient Tip: Made from the dried and ground berries of a wild sumac flower, sumac is a tangy, slightly sour spice that's a staple in Middle Eastern cooking. Its acidic taste is similar to lemon juice and pairs well with salad dressings. You should be able to find sumac in most grocery store spice aisles or online. If you can't find it, you can substitute grated lemon zest.

Per Serving: Calories: 414; Fat: 25g; Carbohydrates: 44g; Fiber: 13g; Sugar: 8g; Protein: 12g; Sodium: 1,243mg

Fiery Curry Pasta Salad

SERVES 4   PREP TIME: 15 MINUTES   COOK TIME: 15 MINUTES
NUT-FREE, SOY-FREE

When I first created this dish, it was a replica of a chicken salad from a favorite childhood restaurant and was not vegan. It then morphed into a vegan chickpea version, a tofu variation, and eventually a plant-based chick'n one. Recently, I got the idea to turn it into a pasta salad and to dial up the heat with hot curry powder. It's creamy, fiery, and delicious. It's also a great canvas for whatever veggies you have hanging around—just add them in.

1 (16-ounce) box uncooked whole-wheat fusilli or penne

2 cups frozen broccoli florets

1 medium carrot, shredded

2 celery stalks, diced

1 green apple, cored and diced

½ small red onion, diced

½ cup unsweetened dried cranberries

¼ cup vegan mayonnaise

Juice of 1 lime

2 tablespoons hot curry powder

1. In a large pot, cook the pasta according to the package directions. During the last 2 minutes of cooking, add the broccoli to the pasta water. Drain, reserving ¼ cup of pasta water. Set aside.

2. Meanwhile, in a large bowl, combine the carrot, celery, apple, onion, and cranberries. Set aside.

3. In a small bowl, whisk together the mayonnaise, lime juice, curry powder, and 2 tablespoons of reserved pasta water to form a sauce. If still too thick, add the remaining 2 tablespoons of pasta water.

4. Add the pasta and broccoli to the large bowl with the veggies, pour the dressing over everything, and toss well to coat before serving.

Variation Tip: If fiery spice isn't your thing, swap the hot curry powder for a mild Madras curry powder. You'll get all the warm, sensuous flavors of curry without the burn.

Per Serving: Calories: 629; Fat: 15g; Carbohydrates: 115g; Fiber: 16g; Sugar: 26g; Protein: 18g; Sodium: 208mg

Not-Tuna Melt

SERVES 4   **PREP TIME:** 20 MINUTES   **COOK TIME:** 5 MINUTES
NUT-FREE, OIL-FREE

Tuna melts were a favorite of mine as a kid. When I became vegan, my goal was to create a delicious vegan tuna spread. And when dairy-free Cheddar slices became mainstream, I recreated the tuna melt. This recipe uses store-bought vegan cheese, such as Daiya or Miyoko's, because it's a comfort food dish and life is about balance. But if you want to avoid it, you can simply put the open-faced sandwich under the broiler to give it that warm, toasty crunch.

1 (15-ounce) can no-salt-added chickpeas, drained and rinsed

1 (15-ounce) can hearts of palm, drained and finely chopped

2 celery stalks, diced

3 scallions, diced

1 large dill pickle, diced, or 1 tablespoon sweet pickle relish

2 tablespoons low-sodium tamari

1 teaspoon yellow mustard

½ teaspoon kelp granules

½ teaspoon kosher salt

½ teaspoon freshly ground black pepper

8 slices sprouted grain or whole-wheat bread

4 slices dairy-free Cheddar cheese

1. Preheat the oven to 450°F. Line a standard baking sheet with parchment paper.

2. In a large bowl, using a fork or potato masher, mash the chickpeas until they're well mashed. Add the hearts of palm and mash until combined.

3. Add the celery, scallions, pickle, tamari, mustard, kelp, salt, and pepper and mix until well combined.

4. Place all 8 slices of bread on the prepared baking sheet. Spread the "tuna" mix evenly on 4 of the slices and top each with a single slice of cheese.

5. Bake for 5 minutes, or until the cheese is melted and the bread is toasted. Remove from the oven and form sandwiches by placing the plain toast on top of the melted cheese. Enjoy warm.

Ingredient Tip: Kelp granules (or flakes) are made from dried seaweed that is crumbled into flakes and used to add a briny, fish-like flavor to vegan dishes. They're naturally low in sodium and full of antioxidants. You can easily find kelp flakes at most health food stores and online, or in the seafood section of many regular grocery stores.

Per Serving: Calories: 415; Fat: 9g; Carbohydrates: 70g; Fiber: 13g; Sugar: 10g; Protein: 17g; Sodium: 1,364mg

Buffalo Smashed Chickpea Sandwich

SERVES 4   PREP TIME: 20 MINUTES
NUT-FREE, OIL-FREE, SOY-FREE

This is my go-to weekday lunch. It's got good heat from the hot sauce (I like Frank's RedHot) that is balanced nicely by the creamy avocado, cool tomatoes, and leafy greens. I make a batch of the Buffalo chickpea spread (through step 2) on Sunday evenings and eat it throughout the week when I need a quick, protein-packed lunch. This spread is also great in a salad or as a snack with your favorite crackers and some cut veggies.

2 (15-ounce) cans no-salt-added chickpeas, drained and rinsed

½ red onion, finely diced

2 celery stalks, finely diced

¼ cup shredded carrots

½ teaspoon kosher salt

½ teaspoon freshly ground black pepper

¼ cup vegan Buffalo hot sauce

6 tablespoons plain hummus, divided, or 4 tablespoons vegan mayonnaise

1 avocado, mashed

8 slices whole-grain bread

Leafy greens of choice

2 beefsteak tomatoes, thickly sliced

1. In a large bowl, using a potato masher or a fork, mash the chickpeas until they're almost flaky in texture and no whole chickpeas remain.

2. Add the red onion, celery, carrots, salt, pepper, hot sauce, and 4 tablespoons of hummus or mayonnaise and mix until thoroughly combined.

3. In a small bowl, mash the avocado and mix it with the remaining 2 tablespoons of hummus. Spread the avocado evenly on all the bread slices. Layer 4 slices with leafy greens.

4. Add about ¼ cup of the chickpea mix to each of the 4 slices, spreading it out evenly over the greens, then top with 2 slices of tomato and another slice of bread. Enjoy immediately.

Per Serving: Calories: 542; Fat: 16g; Carbohydrates: 79g; Fiber: 19g; Sugar: 13g; Protein: 24g; Sodium: 985mg

Jerk Jackfruit Wraps

SERVES 4   PREP TIME: 10 MINUTES   **COOK TIME:** 20 MINUTES
ONE-POT, NUT-FREE, OIL-FREE, SOY-FREE

Jerk is native to Jamaica and involves using either a dry spice mix or a wet marinade made from warm, rich spices, including cinnamon, nutmeg, clove, ginger, allspice, garlic, and scotch bonnet peppers for some fierce heat. It's wonderfully fragrant and pairs well with jackfruit, which has a very meaty consistency. This dish uses a premade wet jerk marinade, such as Eaton's or Grace, but could also be made with a dry jerk seasoning mix and a couple of tablespoons of neutral oil, such as grapeseed.

1 (20-ounce) can young jackfruit packed in water, drained

¼ cup store-bought jerk seasoning sauce

3 cups frozen mango, thawed and diced

1 small red onion, diced

⅛ teaspoon tabasco or other hot sauce

½ cup chopped fresh cilantro or flat-leaf parsley

Juice of 1 lime

¼ teaspoon kosher salt

8 medium or 4 large Bibb lettuce leaves

4 (10-inch) whole-wheat tortillas

1. Heat a large skillet over medium-high heat. Using your fingers, shred the jackfruit and put it in the skillet, along with the jerk seasoning sauce. Cook, stirring frequently, for 15 to 20 minutes, or until the edges caramelize.

2. In a medium bowl, combine the mango, onion, hot sauce, cilantro, lime juice, and salt. Taste and adjust the salt and hot sauce as needed.

3. Divide the lettuce leaves evenly among the 4 tortillas, and top with the jerk jackfruit and mango salsa. Roll up the wrap by first tucking in the sides and then folding over the edge closest to you and rolling up. Cut in half and enjoy.

Variation Tip: Easily make this dish gluten-free by omitting the tortillas and using large lettuce leaves (Bibb or iceberg work best) to make these into lettuce wraps. Alternatively, this dish is lovely served over a bed of crisp greens.

Per Serving: Calories: 335; Fat: 7g; Carbohydrates: 63g; Fiber: 10g; Sugar: 21g; Protein: 7g; Sodium: 790mg

Nashville Hot Tofu Sandwich

SERVES 4   **PREP TIME:** 10 MINUTES   **COOK TIME:** 15 MINUTES
NUT-FREE

This is my 30-minute vegan twist on a Nashville hot chicken sandwich. Typically, the tofu is breaded and deep-fried or baked, but that's a tall task in 30 minutes. This version cooks in less time and still delivers that savory, sweet, flaming-hot flavor that this sandwich is known for. Unlike Buffalo sauce, which is equal parts butter and hot sauce, Nashville hot sauce adds pepper, garlic, paprika, and brown sugar (or agave syrup) to add deep flavor along with the heat. I like to serve half of this sandwich paired with a crisp, fresh salad for a delicious combo meal.

1 (12-ounce) block extra-firm tofu, drained and pressed

2 tablespoons grapeseed oil or extra-virgin olive oil

2 tablespoons vegan butter

⅓ cup hot sauce (I prefer Frank's RedHot)

2 tablespoons brown sugar

2 teaspoons kosher salt

2 teaspoons freshly ground black pepper

1 teaspoon paprika

2 teaspoons garlic powder

2 large hamburger buns or round Italian buns

⅓ cup bread and butter pickles

1. Halve the block of tofu lengthwise so that you have two strips. Cut each strip in half to create four squares.

2. In a large skillet, heat the oil over medium-high heat until it shimmers. Add the tofu squares and cook for 2 to 3 minutes per side, or until golden. Remove the skillet from the heat and set aside. Leave the tofu in the skillet.

3. In a small saucepan over low heat, combine the butter, hot sauce, brown sugar, salt, pepper, paprika, and garlic powder and cook, whisking constantly, until heated through and combined.

4. Add the sauce to the skillet with the tofu and toss to coat. Place two tofu fillets on the bottom half of each bun and drizzle 1 tablespoon of sauce on each. Add the pickles, then cover with the top half of the bun. Serve with the remaining sauce for dipping, if desired.

Cooking Tip: Extra-firm tofu contains the least amount of water of any type of tofu and doesn't require much time or equipment to press. Simply drain the tofu from the package, wrap in a couple of layers of paper towel (or a clean kitchen towel), and press down on it for 1 to 2 minutes to squeeze out any water.

Per Serving: Calories: 319; Fat: 18g; Carbohydrates: 27g; Fiber: 2g; Sugar: 9g; Protein: 13g; Sodium: 1,581mg

Un-Crab Salad Po' Boy

SERVES 4   **PREP TIME:** 20 MINUTES
NUT-FREE

A Po' Boy is a classic Louisiana sandwich typically made with shrimp that is usually breaded and fried and served on a baguette with lettuce, tomato, and a French remoulade sauce. Because vegan shrimp is hard to replicate without using a store-bought product, I'm using an adapted version of my spicy un-crab salad instead and flavoring it with the classic ingredients of remoulade.

1 (12-ounce) block extra-firm tofu, drained and pressed

3 tablespoons vegan mayonnaise

1 tablespoon Dijon mustard

1 teaspoon white vinegar

½ teaspoon Cajun seasoning or Old Bay seasoning

½ teaspoon prepared horseradish

½ to 1 teaspoon sriracha or other hot sauce

4 small French sandwich rolls

½ head lettuce, shredded

2 or 3 tomatoes, sliced ¼-inch thick

1. Using the large grate side of a box grater, shred the tofu and put it in a medium bowl.

2. Add the mayonnaise, mustard, vinegar, Cajun seasoning, horseradish, and sriracha and mix well to combine. Taste and adjust the hot sauce as necessary.

3. Slice each sandwich roll almost all the way through and place a layer of shredded lettuce on each one. Divide the salad evenly among the rolls and top with a layer of sliced tomatoes. Press the top of the bread down gently to compress the sandwich slightly before enjoying.

Variation Tip: If you're looking for a more authentic breaded sandwich, cube the tofu instead of shredding and dredge it in coconut milk, followed by a mix of equal parts fine cornmeal and all-purpose flour and some Cajun seasoning. Bake in the oven at 400°F until crispy, or panfry in oil. Make the remoulade sauce separately, then mix the cooked tofu with the sauce.

Per Serving: Calories: 414; Fat: 15g; Carbohydrates: 52g; Fiber: 6g; Sugar: 6g; Protein: 19g; Sodium: 670mg

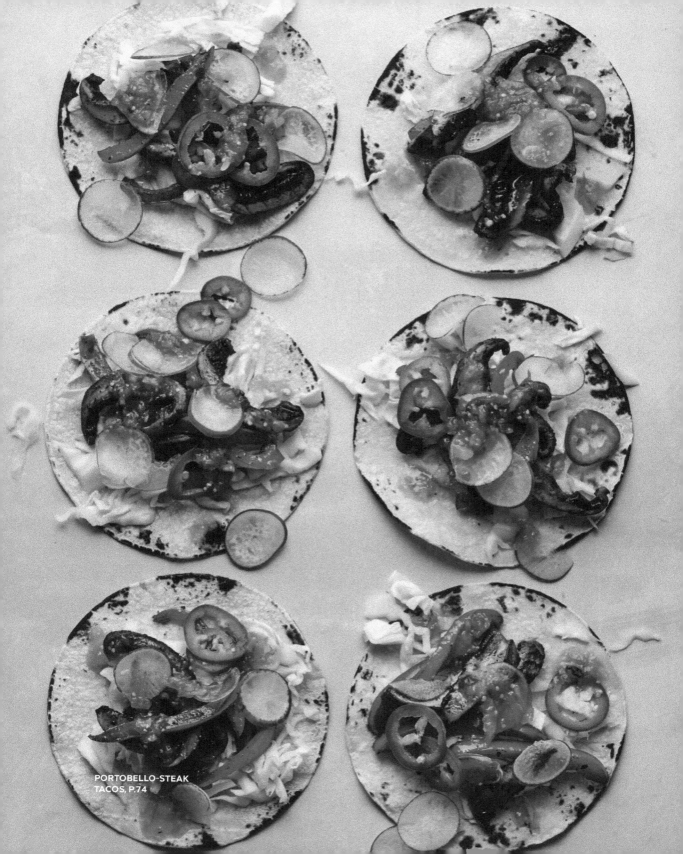

PORTOBELLO-STEAK
TACOS, P.74

5

Hearty Mains

Easy Lahmajoun (Armenian-Style Pizza)   64

Italian-Style Zucchini, Spinach, and Bean Skillet   65

Jeweled Rice   66

Ginger Coconut Tofu with Snap Peas and Cashews   67

Everything Bagel Crusted Tofu Fillets
and Green Beans   68

Spicy Korean-Inspired Barbecue Tofu Bowl   70

Tex-Mex Polenta Bowl   72

Chipotle Sweet Potato and Navy Bean Stew   73

Portobello-Steak Tacos   74

Black Bean and Sweet Potato Enchiladas   75

Tteokbokki (Spicy Korean-Style Rice Cake Stew)   76

Polenta-Stuffed Portobello Stacks   78

Tempeh and Asian Pear Bulgogi   79

Spicy Mixed Bean Jambalaya   80

Unstuffed Cabbage Rolls   81

Easy Lahmajoun (Armenian-Style Pizza)

SERVES 4 PREP TIME: 10 MINUTES COOK TIME: 15 MINUTES
NUT-FREE, OIL-FREE, SOY-FREE

Lahmajoun is a traditional personal-size Armenian-style pizza made with well-spiced ground meat and diced vegetables on top of a homemade dough. I'm giving this version a vegan spin by using mashed chickpeas in place of meat and taking a shortcut for the dough, swapping the dough for flour tortillas, which is a very common American adaptation. You could also use thin pita.

¾ cup no-salt-added canned chickpeas, drained and rinsed

¼ medium yellow onion, finely diced

1 teaspoon jarred minced garlic or 2 garlic cloves, minced

1 cup regular or spicy hummus

2 tablespoons tomato paste

2 tablespoons mild or sweet red pepper paste

1 cup loosely packed fresh flat-leaf parsley, finely chopped

1 teaspoon smoked paprika

1 teaspoon ground cumin

½ teaspoon kosher salt

½ teaspoon freshly ground black pepper

8 (8-inch) whole-wheat flour tortillas

1. Preheat the oven to 400°F. Line two large baking sheets with parchment or aluminum foil.

2. In a large bowl, using a potato masher or a fork, mash the chickpeas into a chunky mashed consistency. Add the onion, garlic, hummus, tomato paste, red pepper paste, parsley, paprika, cumin, salt, and black pepper and mix well to combine.

3. Place 3 tortillas on each prepared baking sheet and spoon about 3 tablespoons of the chickpea mixture onto each one, spreading it evenly almost to the edges. Place both baking sheets in the oven (one on each rack) and bake for 5 to 6 minutes, or until the edges of the tortillas are nicely browned. Repeat with remaining tortillas (working in batches of 3 or less) and serve immediately.

Ingredient Tip: Red pepper paste is a spread made from roasted red bell peppers and is typically mild or sweet. Find it in the condiments or international foods section.

Per Serving (2 pizzas): Calories: 534; Fat: 18g; Carbohydrates: 80g; Fiber: 14g; Sugar: 10g; Protein: 17g; Sodium: 1,893mg

Italian-Style Zucchini, Spinach, and Bean Skillet

SERVES 4 **PREP TIME:** 10 MINUTES **COOK TIME:** 20 MINUTES
ONE-POT, GLUTEN-FREE, NUT-FREE, OIL-FREE, SOY-FREE

This is a wonderfully flavored quick stew that is packed with protein and comes together in minutes. I don't normally use instant rice, but in this dish it helps thicken up the stew and adds bulk with minimal cooking time. I like zucchini and spinach here, but you could use any leftover veggies you have. Just be sure to cut heartier veggies super small so that they cook quickly.

2 tablespoons low-sodium vegetable broth or water, plus 1 cup

½ large yellow onion, diced

1 zucchini, skin on, cut into half-moons

1 (15-ounce) can low-sodium diced tomatoes

1 (15-ounce) can no-salt-added chickpeas, drained and rinsed

1 (15-ounce) can no-salt-added cannellini beans, drained and rinsed

¾ cup uncooked instant rice

1 teaspoon Italian seasoning blend

1 cup marinara sauce

3 cups packed baby spinach

1. Heat a large skillet over medium heat. Combine 2 tablespoons of broth, the onion, and zucchini and cook until soft, about 5 minutes, stirring occasionally.

2. Add the tomatoes with their juices, chickpeas, beans, remaining 1 cup of broth, the rice, and Italian seasoning and bring to a boil over high heat.

3. Reduce the heat to medium-low, cover, and simmer for 8 to 10 minutes, or until the rice is tender. Stir in the marinara sauce and spinach.

4. Remove from the stove and let the residual heat wilt the spinach before serving.

Ingredient Tip: Italian seasoning blend is one of the most common spice blends in your supermarket's spice aisle. Made up of marjoram, basil, oregano, thyme, rosemary, and sage, it's an easy way to add flavor without taking up tons of pantry space or measuring time.

Per Serving: Calories: 335; Fat: 4g; Carbohydrates: 61g; Fiber: 13g; Sugar: 14g; Protein: 15g; Sodium: 483mg

Jeweled Rice

SERVES 4   PREP TIME: 10 MINUTES   COOK TIME: 20 MINUTES
GLUTEN-FREE, SOY-FREE

Jeweled rice is a dish with roots in the Middle East that is traditionally served at weddings and other celebrations. Typically, this is a low-simmering dish with multiple steps, but I've created a shortcut version that is just as bright and beautiful, yet easy enough to get on the table for a weeknight dinner. To give this dish a protein boost, try adding some shelled edamame or roasted tofu cubes.

2 cups uncooked basmati rice

4 cups low-sodium vegetable broth

½ teaspoon ground turmeric

2 tablespoons grapeseed oil or extra-virgin olive oil

½ yellow onion, diced

½ cup shredded carrots

½ teaspoon ground cinnamon

1 teaspoon grated orange zest

½ cup golden raisins

1 cup shelled, roasted, unsalted pistachios

½ cup dried unsweetened cranberries

½ cup pomegranate seeds

1. In a medium pot with a tight-fitting lid, combine the rice, broth, and turmeric and bring to a boil over high heat. Immediately reduce the heat to low, cover, and cook for 15 minutes, or until the rice is tender and the broth is absorbed. Fluff with a fork and set aside.

2. Meanwhile, in a large skillet, heat the oil over medium-high heat. Add the onion and carrots and cook until the onion starts to soften, about 4 minutes. Add the cinnamon and orange zest and cook, stirring constantly, for 1 more minute. Remove from the heat and stir in the golden raisins. Add the cooked rice to the skillet and stir to combine.

3. Spread the rice mixture evenly on a large oval serving platter and top with pistachios, cranberries, and pomegranate seeds.

Per Serving: Calories: 716; Fat: 22g; Carbohydrates: 120g; Fiber: 6g; Sugar: 35g; Protein: 14g; Sodium: 174mg

Ginger Coconut Tofu with Snap Peas and Cashews

SERVES 4 **PREP TIME:** 10 MINUTES **COOK TIME:** 15 MINUTES
GLUTEN-FREE, OIL-FREE

I always have this dish in my rotation. It's delightfully delicious and so easy to make. Snap peas and cashews add great crunch and are easy to just toss in the skillet, but you could use other leftover veggies as well. To keep this dish on the healthier side, I've suggested a light coconut milk, but if you want a luxuriously rich sauce, use full-fat coconut milk instead.

1 (14-ounce) block extra-firm tofu, drained, pressed, and cut into 1-inch cubes

1 tablespoon cornstarch

¼ cup cold water

½ cup light canned coconut milk

3 tablespoons low-sodium tamari

1 teaspoon grated ginger, jarred or fresh

3 tablespoons brown sugar

½ teaspoon sriracha sauce

½ cup unsalted roasted cashews

½ cup sugar snap peas

½ cup unsweetened shredded coconut

1. Preheat the oven to 400°F. Line a standard baking sheet with parchment paper.

2. Place the tofu on the baking sheet in a single layer and put it in the oven during the preheat time. Bake for 10 minutes from the time the oven is fully heated, or until the tofu cubes are lightly golden.

3. Meanwhile, make the sauce. In a medium bowl, whisk together the cornstarch and water until fully dissolved. Add the coconut milk, tamari, ginger, brown sugar, and sriracha and stir to combine.

4. Transfer the sauce to a large skillet over medium-high heat and bring to a simmer, stirring constantly, until the sauce is thick enough to coat the back of a spoon, about 2 minutes. Add the cooked tofu, cashews, and snap peas and toss to combine. Remove from the heat and sprinkle with shredded coconut before serving.

Per Serving: Calories: 303; Fat: 19g; Carbohydrates: 22g; Fiber: 4g; Sugar: 9g; Protein: 15g; Sodium: 568mg

Everything Bagel Crusted Tofu Fillets and Green Beans

SERVES 4 **PREP TIME:** 10 MINUTES **COOK TIME:** 20 MINUTES
GLUTEN-FREE, NUT-FREE, OIL-FREE

Everything bagel seasoning is a delicious mix of white and black sesame seeds, poppy seeds, garlic granules, minced dried onion, and salt. Its origins started with—you guessed it—bagels, but it has become a popular ingredient for all types of dishes. In this recipe, I've paired it with tamari and crushed red pepper flakes to add a delicious crust to baked tofu fillets. The red pepper flakes are of course optional, but they do add a nice heat.

1 (14-ounce) package extra-firm tofu, drained and quickly pressed
¼ cup low-sodium tamari
3 tablespoons cornstarch
¼ cup everything bagel seasoning
½ teaspoon crushed red pepper flakes (optional)

1 pound green beans, ends trimmed
1 teaspoon jarred minced garlic or 2 garlic cloves, minced
1 tablespoon lemon zest
1 tablespoon lemon juice

1. Preheat the oven to 400°F. Line a standard baking sheet with parchment paper.

2. Slice the tofu into ¼-inch fillets and place in a shallow bowl. Pour the tamari over the tofu and let it sit for a minute while you mix the dry seasoning.

3. In another shallow bowl, combine the cornstarch, everything bagel seasoning, and red pepper flakes (if using). Dip each piece of tofu into the seasoning mix, toss to coat, and place on the prepared baking sheet. Bake for 20 minutes, flipping halfway through.

4. Meanwhile, boil a medium pot of water and fill a large bowl with ice water. Add the green beans to the pot of boiling water and cook for 3 minutes, then immediately remove and submerge them in the ice water. This stops the cooking process and retains that bright green color.

5. Heat a large skillet over medium-high heat. Combine the garlic, lemon zest, lemon juice, and green beans and cook, tossing constantly, for 2 to 3 minutes. Remove from the heat and serve with the baked tofu.

Ingredient Tip: Everything bagel seasoning is easy to get at most grocery stores now, but if you can't find it, you can make your own for this dish by combining 2 tablespoons of white sesame seeds, 2 tablespoons of black sesame seeds, 2 tablespoons of poppy seeds, 1 teaspoon of granulated onion, 1 teaspoon of granulated garlic, and ½ teaspoon of kosher salt.

Per Serving: Calories: 237; Fat: 6g; Carbohydrates: 19g; Fiber: 5g; Sugar: 4g; Protein: 15g; Sodium: 1,674mg

Spicy Korean-Inspired Barbecue Tofu Bowl

SERVES 4   **PREP TIME:** 15 MINUTES   **COOK TIME:** 15 MINUTES
GLUTEN-FREE, NUT-FREE

This is by far my favorite #betterthantakeout dish. I typically use tofu here, but if you want a soy-free version you could use jackfruit or steamed broccoli. It is really worth finding genuine gochujang for this recipe. Gochujang is a Korean fermented chili paste that is hot like sriracha, but with much more flavor. It's becoming more popular at regular grocery stores and is widely available at Asian supermarkets and online.

1½ cups uncooked brown basmati rice

3 cups low-sodium vegetable broth

3 tablespoons grapeseed oil or extra-virgin olive oil, divided

1 (14-ounce) package extra-firm tofu

½ red onion, roughly chopped

1 small zucchini, cut into half-moons

1 (8-ounce) can pineapple chunks, drained well

1 teaspoon coconut sugar

2 tablespoons gochujang

⅓ cup vegan barbecue sauce

2 tablespoons low-sodium tamari

2 teaspoons ground ginger

2 teaspoons garlic powder

1. In a medium pot with a tight-fitting lid, combine the rice and broth and bring to a boil over high heat. Reduce the heat to low, cover, and cook for 15 minutes, or until the rice is tender and the broth is absorbed. Fluff with a fork and set aside.

2. Meanwhile, in a large skillet, heat 2 tablespoons of oil over medium-high heat until it shimmers. Add the tofu and cook, tossing occasionally, until crispy and golden on all sides. Remove the tofu from the skillet and place on a plate and cover with foil. Set aside.

3. Return the skillet to the stove and heat the remaining 1 tablespoon of oil. Add the onion and zucchini and cook until crisp-tender, about 4 minutes. Push them to the side of the skillet, add the pineapple and sugar in the middle, and cook for 2 minutes, stirring constantly, until soft and lightly caramelized. Remove the skillet from the heat. Return the tofu to the skillet and toss to combine. Cover and set aside.

4. To make the sauce, in a medium bowl, combine the gochujang, barbecue sauce, tamari, ginger, and garlic powder and whisk well. Pour over the tofu and vegetables and stir to combine.

5. Divide the rice evenly among four serving bowls and top with tofu and vegetables. Enjoy.

Ingredient Tip: Many store-bought brands of barbecue sauce are naturally vegan, making them a great way to add smoky, bold barbecue flavor to your dishes. For this recipe, I like to use Sweet Baby Ray's or Annie's Naturals Organic Original BBQ.

Per Serving: Calories: 528; Fat: 19g; Carbohydrates: 76g; Fiber: 6g; Sugar: 17g; Protein: 19g; Sodium: 764mg

Tex-Mex Polenta Bowl

SERVES 4   PREP TIME: 10 MINUTES   **COOK TIME:** 20 MINUTES
GLUTEN-FREE, NUT-FREE, OIL-FREE, SOY-FREE

I absolutely love the contrast in colors, textures, and flavors of this dish. Polenta is a great alternative to the usual rice or pasta, and it works so well with Tex-Mex flavors. This bowl gets a bright punch of flavor from homemade pico de gallo, which is a fresh, chunky salsa made from tomatoes, onions, cilantro, lime, and salt. Adding jalapeño peppers gives it a nice heat.

4 cups low-sodium vegetable broth

1 cup dry cornmeal

1 teaspoon ground cumin

2 tablespoons nutritional yeast

½ teaspoon kosher salt

1 cup grape tomatoes, halved

½ small red onion, diced

2 tablespoons finely chopped fresh flat-leaf parsley or cilantro

Juice of 1 lime

1 (15-ounce) can no-salt-added black or pinto beans, drained and rinsed

1 large avocado, cubed

1 jalapeño pepper, cut into rings

1. In a medium saucepan over high heat, bring the broth to a boil, then gradually whisk in the cornmeal. Reduce the heat to low and stir in the cumin and nutritional yeast. Cook, stirring occasionally, until the cornmeal is thick and creamy, about 20 minutes. Remove from the heat and whisk in the salt.

2. To make the pico de gallo, in a small bowl, combine the tomatoes, onion, parsley, and lime juice. Set aside.

3. Divide the polenta among four bowls. Top each with about ¼ cup of beans and garnish with pico de gallo, avocado, and jalapeño peppers before serving.

Ingredient Tip: In a hot pepper, most of the heat is in the seeds. Remove the seeds from your jalapeño pepper for less heat.

Per Serving: Calories: 370; Fat: 9g; Carbohydrates: 62g; Fiber: 16g; Sugar: 5g; Protein: 14g; Sodium: 288mg

Chipotle Sweet Potato and Navy Bean Stew

SERVES 4   PREP TIME: 10 MINUTES   **COOK TIME:** 20 MINUTES
ONE-POT, GLUTEN-FREE, NUT-FREE, OIL-FREE, SOY-FREE

This is a warm, comforting winter dish that is easy to make and so customizable. Chipotle pepper and cumin add mild heat and warm flavors that pair so well with roasted tomatoes and sweet potatoes. I like to use navy beans in this dish, but any bean or chickpeas work well, too. Precut sweet potatoes (either frozen or fresh) drastically reduce your prep time for this recipe.

3 tablespoons low-sodium vegetable broth, plus 3 cups

½ medium yellow onion, diced

1 teaspoon jarred minced garlic or 2 garlic cloves, minced

1 tablespoon chipotle powder

½ teaspoon ground cumin

1 (15-ounce) can no-salt-added navy beans, drained and rinsed

2 cups chopped frozen or fresh sweet potatoes

1 (15-ounce) can fire-roasted crushed or diced tomatoes

2 cups baby spinach

1. In a large pot, heat 3 tablespoons of broth over medium heat. Add the onion and cook for 3 to 4 minutes, or until softened.

2. Add the garlic, chipotle powder, and cumin and cook, stirring constantly, for 30 seconds, or until the spices are fragrant. Add the beans, sweet potatoes, tomatoes with their juices, and remaining 3 cups of vegetable broth and bring to a boil. Reduce the heat to a simmer and cook for 15 minutes, or until the sweet potatoes are tender.

3. Remove the pot from the heat, then add the spinach and stir until it's wilted. Serve warm.

Per Serving: Calories: 277; Fat: 1g; Carbohydrates: 57g; Fiber: 15g; Sugar: 10g; Protein: 11g; Sodium: 458mg

Portobello-Steak Tacos

SERVES 4   **PREP TIME:** 15 MINUTES   **COOK TIME:** 15 MINUTES
GLUTEN-FREE, NUT-FREE

Taco Tuesday just got a major upgrade. Portobello mushrooms give this dish an intensely meaty flavor and consistency and are delicious paired with crunchy cabbage, tangy salsa verde, and the briny heat of pickled jalapeños. Occasionally, if I have vegan sour cream on hand, I like to mix ¼ cup with the juice of half a lime and some chopped fresh cilantro to make a crema sauce to drizzle on top.

5 portobello mushroom caps, sliced about
  ½-inch thick

1 red bell pepper, seeded and cut into
  ¼-inch strips

1 tablespoon low-sodium tamari

1 teaspoon chili powder

2 tablespoons grapeseed oil or extra-virgin
  olive oil

1 (7-ounce) bag shredded cabbage or
  coleslaw mix

12 small corn tortillas, warmed in the oven or
  microwaved in a damp towel

4 radishes, thinly sliced

⅓ cup pickled jalapeño peppers

½ cup store-bought salsa verde

1. In a large bowl, combine the mushrooms, bell pepper, tamari, and chili powder and toss to coat.

2. In a large skillet, heat the oil over medium-high heat until it shimmers. Working in two or three batches and being careful not to overcrowd the skillet, add the mushrooms and bell peppers and cook for 3 to 4 minutes, or until the mushrooms are browned. Transfer to a plate, cover with foil, and repeat with the remaining mushrooms and bell peppers.

3. Assemble the tacos by dividing the cabbage evenly among all 12 tortillas. Top with the mushrooms and peppers, garnish with radishes and pickled jalapeños, and drizzle with salsa verde before enjoying.

Cooking Tip: Instead of cooking on the stovetop, you can turn this into a sheet pan dish by mixing the mushrooms, bell pepper, oil, tamari, and chili powder together and then transferring everything to a large parchment-lined rimmed baking sheet. Bake at 400°F for 15 to 20 minutes.

Per Serving (3 tacos): Calories: 277; Fat: 10g; Carbohydrates: 44g; Fiber: 9g; Sugar: 8g; Protein: 8g; Sodium: 771mg

Black Bean and Sweet Potato Enchiladas

SERVES 4   PREP TIME: 10 MINUTES   **COOK TIME:** 20 MINUTES
ONE-POT, NUT-FREE, OIL-FREE, SOY-FREE

What I love most about this dish is that it's a great canvas for whatever you've got lying around the house. In fact, I created it by rummaging through the refrigerator one day looking for dinner inspiration. You can swap the sweet potato for butternut squash or another veggie, use any type of bean you have in the pantry, or bulk it up by adding leftover cooked rice.

2 tablespoons slow-sodium vegetable broth or water, plus 1 cup

1 medium yellow onion, diced

1 teaspoon jarred minced garlic or 2 garlic cloves, minced

1 tablespoon chili powder

1 teaspoon ground cumin

¼ teaspoon ground cinnamon

1 (16-ounce) bag frozen diced sweet potatoes

1 (15-ounce) can no-salt-added black beans, drained and rinsed

1½ cups store-bought enchilada sauce, divided

1 (12-ounce) can no-salt-added corn, drained

8 (10-inch) whole-wheat flour tortillas

1. In a large skillet, heat 2 tablespoons of broth over medium heat until it reaches just below a simmer. Add the onion and cook for 5 minutes, or until soft. Add the garlic, chili powder, cumin, and cinnamon and cook, stirring constantly, for 30 seconds.

2. Add the sweet potatoes, beans, remaining 1 cup of vegetable broth, and ½ cup of enchilada sauce. Simmer for 10 to 15 minutes, stirring occasionally, until most of the broth has been absorbed. Remove from the heat and stir in the corn.

3. Divide the filling equally among the tortillas, roll up, and top with the remaining 1 cup of enchilada sauce before serving.

Per Serving (2 enchiladas): Calories: 705; Fat: 12g; Carbohydrates: 132g; Fiber: 22g; Sugar: 15g; Protein: 23g; Sodium: 1,661mg

Tteokbokki (Spicy Korean-Style Rice Cake Stew)

SERVES 6 **PREP TIME:** 10 MINUTES **COOK TIME:** 15 MINUTES
GLUTEN-FREE, NUT-FREE

I am completely obsessed with this dish. I make it at least once a week—especially in the winter when it's cold outside and I'm looking for something warm and comforting. Tteokbokki is a popular Korean dish made from glutinous rice cakes, spicy Korean fermented chili paste (gochujang), and basically whatever vegetables you have on hand. Many versions include shredded vegan cheese, which I highly recommend for adding that extra layer of chewy, rich texture.

2 cups water

¼ cup gochujang paste

2 tablespoons low-sodium tamari

2 tablespoons pure maple syrup

2 tablespoons grapeseed oil or extra-virgin olive oil

½ medium yellow onion, cut into half-moons

1 carrot, peeled and cut into half-moons

½ bell pepper (any color), seeded and diced

1 (2-pound) bag Korean rice cakes, sticks, or tubes

4 scallions, diced

1 teaspoon sesame oil

1 cup shredded vegan cheese (optional)

Sesame seeds, for garnish

1. In a small bowl, whisk together the water, gochujang, tamari, and maple syrup. Set aside.

2. In a large skillet, heat the grapeseed oil over medium heat. Add the onion, carrot, and bell pepper and cook until soft, about 5 minutes. Add the sauce mix from step 1 and, keeping the skillet over medium heat, bring to a boil.

3. Add the rice cakes and stir to coat. Cook until the rice cakes are soft, 5 to 7 minutes, depending on whether you're using refrigerated or frozen cakes.

4. Once soft, stir in the scallions and sesame oil. Top with shredded cheese (if using), cover, and cook for 5 minutes, or until cheese is all melted. Garnish with sesame seeds before serving.

Ingredient Tip: Topokki, or glutinous rice cakes, are a specialty ingredient worth looking for. Available in tube, stick, or cake form, they are a very dense, chewy rice cake used in Korean cooking that are sold either refrigerated (fresh) or frozen. Despite being called "glutinous rice," topokki should be gluten-free—just read the labels carefully before using if gluten is an issue. Both topokki and gochujang can be found in Asian supermarkets.

Per Serving: Calories: 219; Fat: 7g; Carbohydrates: 39g; Fiber: 3g; Sugar: 10g; Protein: 5g; Sodium: 1,338mg

Polenta-Stuffed Portobello Stacks

SERVES 4   **PREP TIME:** 10 MINUTES   **COOK TIME:** 20 MINUTES
ONE-POT, GLUTEN-FREE, NUT-FREE, OIL-FREE, SOY-FREE

This is an elegant, restaurant-quality dish that is really easy to make but looks like you spent forever in the kitchen. To prepare your portobellos, remove the stem and carefully scrape out the gills from the inside, then use a slightly damp paper towel to gently clean the outside of the cap. Never run mushrooms directly under water as they will absorb it like a sponge, which will affect both texture and taste when cooked.

4 large portobello mushrooms, stemmed and gills removed

2 teaspoons jarred minced garlic or 4 garlic cloves, minced

2 tablespoons chopped fresh basil or 1 tablespoon dried basil

½ teaspoon kosher salt

½ teaspoon freshly ground black pepper

1 tablespoon balsamic vinegar or red wine vinegar

8 (1-inch-thick) slices ready-to-eat polenta

1 large tomato, beefsteak or heirloom, cut into 4 (1-inch-thick) slices

½ cup nutritional yeast, divided

1. Preheat the oven to 400°F.

2. Place the mushrooms in a 9-by-13 baking dish, gill-side up.

3. In a small bowl, combine the garlic, basil, salt, pepper, and vinegar and divide equally among the mushrooms. Layer 2 polenta slices on top of each mushroom so that they overlap slightly and cover the entire mushroom surface. Top each with a tomato slice and 2 tablespoons of nutritional yeast.

4. Bake for 20 to 25 minutes, or until the mushrooms are tender. Serve warm.

Cooking Tip: Ready-to-eat polenta is typically sold in an 18-ounce tube. You won't need the entire tube for this recipe, but you can use up the leftovers to make a delicious breakfast sandwich. Slice the remaining polenta into ½-inch-thick slices and panfry in a little vegan butter along with some nutritional yeast, onion powder, and black salt (kala namak). Serve on a toasted English muffin with your favorite dairy-free cheese or vegan sausage.

Per Serving: Calories: 214; Fat: 1g; Carbohydrates: 40g; Fiber: 12g; Sugar: 4g; Protein: 13g; Sodium: 576mg

Tempeh and Asian Pear Bulgogi

SERVES 4   PREP TIME: 25 MINUTES   COOK TIME: 5 MINUTES
GLUTEN-FREE, NUT-FREE

Bulgogi (Korean marinated beef) was always a pre-vegan favorite of mine, and I've worked for a long time to create a good vegan version that would satisfy my craving. This dish uses Asian pears, which have a very crisp texture and light flavor, like a cross between a pear and an apple, and are often available at grocery stores. If you can't find them, you can swap them for Bartlett or other firm pears. Bulgogi is often served with rice, so I recommend making a pot of basmati or brown rice (or quinoa) to go alongside this dish.

3 tablespoons low-sodium tamari

2 tablespoons mirin or dry white wine, or
  1 tablespoon rice wine vinegar

1 tablespoon coconut sugar

1 tablespoon sesame oil

1 teaspoon jarred minced garlic or 2 garlic
  cloves, minced

1 teaspoon fresh or jarred minced ginger

4 scallions, diced, plus more for garnish

1 (7-ounce) package tempeh strips, halved

½ Asian pear, peeled and grated

1 tablespoon sesame seeds

1. In a large bowl, whisk together the tamari, mirin, sugar, oil, garlic, ginger, and scallions. Add the tempeh and grated pear and let stand for 15 minutes.

2. Heat a dry, large skillet over medium-high heat until it's hot. (Test the skillet by adding a drop of water; if it sizzles and evaporates, the skillet is ready.)

3. Heat the tempeh and pear mixture, including all the marinade, and cook, stirring frequently, for 3 to 5 minutes, or until most of the sauce is reduced.

4. Garnish with sesame seeds and extra scallions before serving.

Variation Tip: If you'd like to steer away from soy products, you can swap the tempeh in this recipe for jackfruit. Simply drain and shred the contents of 1 (14-ounce) can of jackfruit into the marinade along with the pear and cook as directed.

Per Serving: Calories: 183; Fat: 8g; Carbohydrates: 17g; Fiber: 5g; Sugar: 9g; Protein: 10g; Sodium: 538mg

Spicy Mixed Bean Jambalaya

SERVES 6   **PREP TIME:** 5 MINUTES   **COOK TIME:** 25 MINUTES
ONE-POT, FREEZER-FRIENDLY, GLUTEN-FREE, NUT-FREE, OIL-FREE, SOY-FREE

This is the dish that keeps on giving. It's perfect for feeding a hungry crowd for dinner, and it makes the perfect cook-once-eat-all-week lunch on its own, on a salad, or in a wrap. Typically made with meat and seafood, I'm using hearty kidney and pinto beans to give this Creole classic a vegan makeover. Occasionally, if I'm making this dish for a special event, I'll add store-bought vegan sausage, too.

3 cups plus 2 tablespoons low-sodium vegetable broth

1 (14-ounce) can diced tomatoes

1 teaspoon sweet paprika

1 teaspoon chili powder

½ teaspoon dried oregano

½ teaspoon garlic powder

2 cups uncooked basmati rice

1 (14-ounce) bag frozen diced bell peppers and onions

1 (14-ounce) can no-salt-added can red kidney beans, drained and rinsed

1 (14-ounce) can no-salt-added pinto beans, drained and rinsed

1 (12-ounce) can no-salt-added corn, drained

1 to 2 teaspoons hot sauce

1. In a large skillet with a tight-fitting lid, combine the vegetable broth, tomatoes with their juices, paprika, chili powder, oregano, and garlic powder and bring to a boil. Immediately reduce the heat to low. Add the basmati rice and bell pepper and onion mix and simmer, covered, for 20 minutes, or until the rice is fully cooked.

2. Remove from the heat and stir in the kidney beans, pinto beans, corn, and hot sauce to taste. Serve.

Per Serving: Calories: 420; Fat: 2g; Carbohydrates: 88g; Fiber: 9g; Sugar: 9g; Protein: 15g; Sodium: 230mg

Unstuffed Cabbage Rolls

SERVES 6   PREP TIME: 10 MINUTES   **COOK TIME:** 20 MINUTES
GLUTEN-FREE, NUT-FREE, OIL-FREE

My maternal grandfather was Polish, and cabbage rolls were a very big part of his upbringing. While I absolutely love eating authentic homemade rolls, I don't often have the time (or patience) to make them. That's why I love this dish. It's got all the great cabbage roll flavors, but in a deconstructed, 30-minute format. For a truly authentic experience, you could add cooked vegan crumbles, like Beyond or Impossible, but they contain a lot of oil, so use sparingly.

1 cup uncooked basmati rice

2 cups low-sodium vegetable broth or water

1 (28-ounce) can crushed tomatoes

1 (14-ounce) can diced tomatoes, with their liquid

1 tablespoon coconut sugar

2 teaspoons low-sodium tamari

1 teaspoon paprika

1 teaspoon caraway seeds

½ teaspoon cayenne pepper

½ teaspoon kosher salt

½ teaspoon freshly ground black pepper

1 (14-ounce) bag frozen diced bell peppers and onions

1 (14-ounce) bag shredded cabbage or coleslaw mix

1. In a medium pot with a tight-fitting lid, combine the rice and vegetable broth. Bring to a boil over high heat, then immediately reduce the heat to low and cook, covered, for 15 minutes, or until the rice is tender and the broth is absorbed. Remove from the heat and set aside.

2. Meanwhile, in a large stockpot or Dutch oven, combine the crushed and diced tomatoes with their juices, coconut sugar, tamari, paprika, caraway seeds, cayenne pepper, salt, and black pepper and bring to a boil. Stir in the bell pepper and onion mix and cabbage, reduce the heat to a simmer, and cook, covered, for 20 minutes, or until the cabbage is soft.

3. Remove from the heat and stir in the cooked rice. Enjoy.

Per Serving: Calories: 220; Fat: 1g; Carbohydrates: 48g; Fiber: 7g; Sugar: 14g; Protein: 7g; Sodium: 618mg

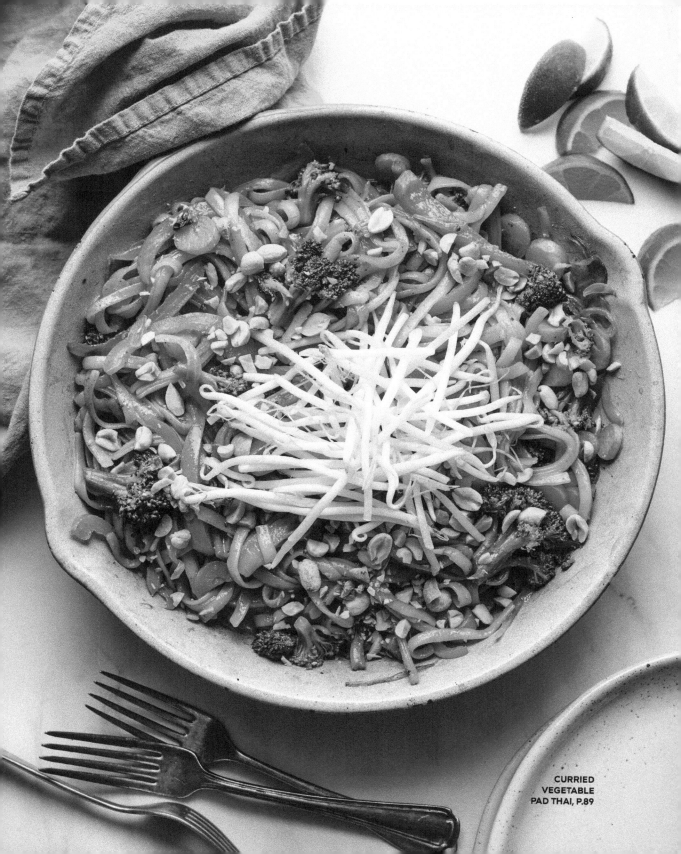

CURRIED
VEGETABLE
PAD THAI, P.89

6

Pasta & Noodles

Edamame Noodle Salad   84

Bruschetta Spaghetti   85

Japchae (Korean-Style Mixed Vegetables
and Glass Noodles)   86

Mediterranean-Inspired White Bean
and Olive Pasta Salad   87

Japanese-Style Mixed Vegetable Noodles   88

Curried Vegetable Pad Thai   89

Penne Arrabbiata with Eggplant   90

Spicy Sesame Broad Rice Noodles   92

Lemon Mushroom Orzo with Spinach and Peas   93

Pasta e Ceci (Italian-Style Chickpea and Pasta Stew)   94

Sun-Dried Tomato and Roasted
Red Pepper Fettuccine Alfredo   96

Creamy Pumpkin Penne   97

Linguini with Artichokes in Lemon Dill Sauce   98

Fusilli with Butter Chicken Sauce and Cherry Tomatoes   99

15-Minute White Mac and "Cheese" with Broccoli   100

Edamame Noodle Salad

SERVES 6 **PREP TIME:** 10 MINUTES   **COOK TIME:** 10 MINUTES
NUT-FREE, OIL-FREE

This is a wonderfully bright, fresh salad that plays on the flavors of teriyaki udon noodles you might find at a Japanese restaurant. Edamame, carrots, and bean sprouts give this dish wonderful texture and crunch, and the dressing adds a punchy, sweet, and nutty flavor thanks to the addition of tahini. Try adding thinly sliced snow peas or shaved Brussels sprouts for more flavor and texture.

8 ounces uncooked udon noodles

2 cups frozen shelled unsalted edamame

5 tablespoons water, divided

3 tablespoons tahini

3 tablespoons low-sodium tamari

3 tablespoons rice wine vinegar

1 teaspoon pure maple syrup

1 teaspoon minced ginger, jarred or fresh

1 cup shredded carrots

2 cups bean sprouts

2 tablespoons sesame seeds

1. Bring a large pot of water to a boil over high heat and cook the udon noodles according to the package directions. Drain and transfer to a large bowl.

2. Meanwhile, in a microwave-safe bowl, combine the edamame and 3 tablespoons of water. Microwave for 3 minutes, then drain and add them to the cooked noodles.

3. In a medium bowl, combine the tahini, tamari, vinegar, remaining 2 tablespoons of water, the maple syrup, and ginger and whisk to form a dressing.

4. Add the dressing, carrots, and bean sprouts to the bowl with the noodles and edamame, tossing well to combine. Sprinkle with sesame seeds before serving.

Per Serving: Calories: 289; Fat: 9g; Carbohydrates: 39g; Fiber: 9g; Sugar: 8g; Protein: 16g; Sodium: 809mg

Bruschetta Spaghetti

SERVES 4 **PREP TIME:** 20 MINUTES **COOK TIME:** 10 MINUTES
NUT-FREE, OIL-FREE, SOY-FREE

This dish combines two of my loves: bruschetta topping and pasta. The combination of tomatoes and fresh basil in this recipe imparts a fresh, bright flavor. You can bump up the veggie content by adding your favorite vegetables. Broccoli is my go-to with pasta. I add a cup or two of frozen broccoli florets to the boiling pasta for the last 2 minutes of cooking time, then strain everything together.

8 ounces uncooked whole-wheat spaghetti

6 plum or Roma tomatoes, seeded and diced

½ cup chopped fresh basil

½ teaspoon crushed red pepper flakes

2 tablespoons jarred minced garlic, or
   4 garlic cloves, minced

½ teaspoon kosher salt

½ teaspoon freshly ground black pepper

3 tablespoons nutritional yeast

1. Bring a large pot of water to a boil over high heat and cook the pasta according to the package directions. Drain and place the pasta back in the pot.

2. Meanwhile, make the bruschetta topping. In a large bowl, combine the tomatoes, basil, red pepper flakes, garlic, salt, and black pepper and toss to combine.

3. When the pasta is done, add the bruschetta topping and the nutritional yeast to the pot and toss to combine. Serve warm.

Variation Tip: Try swapping out the whole-wheat pasta for fresh or frozen spiralized butternut squash or zucchini noodles. Simply steam the spirals according to the package directions, then top with the bruschetta topping and nutritional yeast.

Per Serving: Calories: 244; Fat: 1g; Carbohydrates: 49g; Fiber: 7g; Sugar: 2g; Protein: 12g; Sodium: 151mg

Japchae (Korean-Style Mixed Vegetables and Glass Noodles)

SERVES 5　**PREP TIME:** 20 MINUTES　**COOK TIME:** 10 MINUTES
GLUTEN-FREE, NUT-FREE

Japchae is a very popular, slightly sweet stir-fried noodle and vegetable dish. Japchae literally means "mixed vegetables," and this dish is a great canvas for whatever veggies you've got on hand. Glass noodles are made from sweet potatoes and become clear when cooked, hence their name. They don't require much cooking time, which makes them great for weeknight meals.

6 ounces uncooked sweet potato noodles (also called glass or japchae noodles)

1 tablespoon grapeseed oil or extra-virgin olive oil

½ yellow onion, thinly sliced

1 red bell pepper, seeded and thinly sliced

1 zucchini, cut into half-moons

½ cup cremini mushrooms, thinly sliced

¼ cup low-sodium tamari

1 tablespoon sesame oil

¼ cup brown coconut sugar

1 heaping teaspoon jarred minced garlic, or 3 garlic cloves, minced

½ teaspoon freshly ground black pepper

1. Bring a large pot of water to a boil over high heat and cook the noodles according to the package directions. Drain and run under cold water. Set aside.

2. Meanwhile, in a large skillet, heat the grapeseed oil over medium-high heat until it shimmers. Add the onion, bell pepper, zucchini, and mushrooms and cook, stirring occasionally, for 5 minutes, or until the vegetables soften.

3. In a small bowl, combine the tamari, sesame oil, sugar, garlic, and black pepper. Add the noodles and sauce to the skillet with the vegetables and cook for 2 minutes, tossing constantly, until the noodles are well coated. Serve immediately.

Cooking Tip: To save on prep time, I like to use precut stir-fry vegetables from my grocer's produce section. Most grocery stores offer fresh precut vegetables on their own or in combination packs. Look for a veggie stir-fry package, which should contain most of the veggies listed above.

Per Serving: Calories: 232; Fat: 6g; Carbohydrates: 44g; Fiber: 2g; Sugar: 13g; Protein: 3g; Sodium: 575mg

Mediterranean-Inspired White Bean and Olive Pasta Salad

SERVES 6 PREP TIME: 15 MINUTES **COOK TIME:** 15 MINUTES
NUT-FREE, SOY-FREE

Growing up, I always thought pasta salad had to be cold and full of mayonnaise. This version is the complete opposite. Tricolor veggie-infused pasta, lots of fresh chopped vegetables, and a light dressing make this a definite palate-pleaser. It's delicious both warm or cold, and it travels well, making it a great take-along dish.

1 (12-ounce) box uncooked tricolor veggie fusilli

1 cup grape tomatoes, halved

1 seedless cucumber, chopped

1 yellow bell pepper, seeded and chopped

½ cup jarred roasted red peppers, chopped

7 ounces quartered artichoke hearts, drained

1 (15-ounce) can no-salt-added navy or cannellini beans, drained and rinsed

2 tablespoons extra-virgin olive oil

Juice of 1 lemon

1 tablespoon Italian seasoning blend

½ teaspoon kosher salt

½ teaspoon freshly ground black pepper

½ cup pitted whole kalamata olives

1. Bring a large pot of water to a boil over high heat and cook the pasta according to the package directions. Drain and place in a large bowl. Add the tomatoes, cucumber, bell pepper, roasted red peppers, artichokes, and beans.

2. In a small jar with a tight-fitting lid, combine the oil, lemon juice, Italian seasoning, salt, and black pepper. Close the jar and shake to combine. Pour over the pasta and vegetables and toss to combine. Garnish with kalamata olives before serving.

Per Serving: Calories: 375; Fat: 8g; Carbohydrates: 66g; Fiber: 12g; Sugar: 4g; Protein: 14g; Sodium: 373mg

Japanese-Style Mixed Vegetable Noodles

SERVES 6   PREP TIME: 5 MINUTES   COOK TIME: 10 MINUTES
ONE-POT, NUT-FREE, OIL-FREE

I guarantee you can't get takeout as quickly as you can get this meal on the table. It's about as low-fuss as you can get, but full of flavor. Frozen mixed vegetables are the key to getting this dish done in under 20 minutes. I like to use a vegetable medley like stir-fry or Asian medley (Birds Eye and Green Giant both make excellent options) that can cook in the same pot as the pasta.

1 (16-ounce) package uncooked whole-wheat linguine
1 (12-ounce) bag vegetable medley or Asian medley frozen vegetables
2 tablespoons brown coconut sugar

4 tablespoons low-sodium tamari
1 tablespoon vegetarian hoisin or teriyaki sauce
3 scallions, diced
1 tablespoon sesame seeds

1. Bring a large pot of water to a boil over high heat and cook the linguini according to the package instructions. During the last 2 minutes of cooking, add the frozen vegetables. Drain and return the noodles and veggies to the pot, but keep it off the heat.

2. In a small bowl, whisk together the sugar, tamari, and hoisin sauce. Pour over the noodles and vegetables and toss to coat. The residual heat from the noodles will warm the sauce.

3. Divide into bowls and garnish with scallions and sesame seeds to serve.

Variation Tip: This dish also works well with spiralized zucchini noodles or glass noodles (sweet potato or japchae noodles) if you're looking for a gluten-free, veg-forward substitute for regular pasta.

Per Serving: Calories: 326; Fat: 3g; Carbohydrates: 66g; Fiber: 9g; Sugar: 9g; Protein: 14g; Sodium: 529mg

Curried Vegetable Pad Thai

SERVES 4   **PREP TIME:** 10 MINUTES   **COOK TIME:** 10 MINUTES
GLUTEN-FREE

It's pretty much a given that if I'm at a Thai restaurant or ordering takeout, I'm getting Pad Thai. It's my old reliable, and it never disappoints. One day, my husband convinced me to try something new, so I ordered Curry Pad Thai, and I was smitten with the way the fragrant, mild curry powder flavor played so well with the salty, sweet, and sour notes of Pad Thai. It's become my new favorite, and I'm sure it will be yours, too.

6 ounces uncooked medium-width rice noodles

1 cup frozen broccoli florets

1 cup frozen sliced carrots

3 tablespoons low-sodium tamari

4 teaspoons rice vinegar

2 tablespoons pure maple syrup or agave syrup

1 tablespoon mild yellow curry powder

1 tablespoon grapeseed oil or extra-virgin olive oil

½ red onion, thinly sliced

1 red bell pepper, seeded and thinly sliced

2 cups bean sprouts

¼ cup chopped, roasted, unsalted peanuts

1 lime, cut into wedges

1. Bring a large pot of water to a boil over high heat and cook the rice noodles according to the package directions. During the last 2 minutes of cooking, add the broccoli and carrots. Strain and run under cold water to stop the cooking process and to keep the noodles from sticking. Set aside.

2. Meanwhile, in a small bowl, whisk together the tamari, rice vinegar, maple syrup, and curry powder. Set aside.

3. In a large skillet, heat the oil over medium-high heat until it shimmers. Add the onion and bell pepper and cook until just softened, about 4 minutes. Add the noodles, broccoli, carrots, and sauce and toss to combine. Remove from the heat and top with the bean sprouts and peanuts. Divide among four bowls and serve with lime wedges.

Per Serving: Calories: 333; Fat: 9g; Carbohydrates: 56g; Fiber: 7g; Sugar: 12g; Protein: 10g; Sodium: 645mg

Penne Arrabbiata with Eggplant

SERVES 6   **PREP TIME:** 10 MINUTES   **COOK TIME:** 20 MINUTES
NUT-FREE, SOY-FREE

Penne arrabbiata literally means "angry pasta" in Italian, which is appropriate since it's a fiery hot dish that is bright red. It's my go-to pasta dish whenever we eat out, mostly because it's almost always guaranteed to be vegan and I love a good spicy tomato sauce. I've paired this dish with Japanese eggplant, a long, narrow purple eggplant with a thin skin and creamy flesh. It's less acidic than traditional eggplant and has a sweeter flavor. You can find Japanese eggplant in the produce section of most grocery stores.

1 (12-ounce) box uncooked whole-wheat or tricolor penne rigate

2 tablespoons grapeseed or extra-virgin olive oil, divided

2 small Japanese eggplants, cut into ¾-inch cubes

1 (28-ounce) can crushed tomatoes

1 teaspoon jarred minced garlic, or 2 garlic cloves, minced

½ to 1 teaspoon crushed red pepper flakes

½ teaspoon Italian seasoning blend

2 tablespoons nutritional yeast

1. Bring a large pot of water to a boil over high heat and cook the pasta according to the package directions. Drain, reserving ½ cup of pasta water.

2. In a large skillet, heat 1 tablespoon of oil over medium-high heat until it shimmers. Add half the eggplant and cook, tossing occasionally, until tender, about 4 minutes. Transfer to a plate. Then add the remaining 1 tablespoon of oil and repeat with the remaining eggplant.

3. Return the skillet to medium heat and add the crushed tomatoes with their juices, garlic, red pepper flakes, and Italian seasoning and cook for 5 minutes, or until the sauce thickens slightly.

4. Add the pasta, reserved pasta water, and cooked eggplant to the skillet and cook for 1 minute, tossing to coat in the sauce. Remove from the heat and sprinkle with nutritional yeast before serving.

Cooking Tip: Eggplant has a high water content, and if you overcrowd the skillet it will just steam and get soggy. By cooking the eggplant in two batches, it turns out more panfried as opposed to mushy.

Per Serving: Calories: 337; Fat: 7g; Carbohydrates: 61g; Fiber: 12g; Sugar: 13g; Protein: 13g; Sodium: 267mg

Spicy Sesame Broad Rice Noodles

SERVES 4 **PREP TIME:** 10 MINUTES **COOK TIME:** 10 MINUTES
GLUTEN-FREE, NUT-FREE, OIL-FREE

My kids call this dish "slurpy noodles," and with good reason. It's made from wide rice noodles that are coated in a deliciously pungent hot sauce until they're nice and slippery. My kids have contests to see who can slurp the longest noodle. (Spoiler alert: The 11-year-old always wins over her little sister.) When I make this for them, I dial down the hot sauce a bit, but if it's just the grown-ups eating, the hotter the better!

10 ounces uncooked broad rice noodles

1 cup frozen sliced carrots

1 cup frozen broccoli florets

1 bunch asparagus, ends trimmed, cut into
   2-inch pieces

1/4 cup vegetarian hoisin sauce

1/2 cup low-sodium tamari

1/4 cup water

1 to 2 teaspoons sriracha or other chili paste

2 teaspoons cornstarch

4 scallions, sliced on the diagonal

2 tablespoons sesame seeds

1. Bring a large pot of water to a boil over high heat and cook the rice noodles according to the package directions. During the last 3 minutes of cooking, add the carrots, broccoli, and asparagus. Drain and return to the pot, but keep it off the heat.

2. Meanwhile, in a small pot, whisk together the hoisin sauce, tamari, water, sriracha, and cornstarch over medium heat, until cornstarch is absorbed and the sauce starts to thicken slightly. Remove from the heat and add to the noodles and vegetables. Toss well to coat.

3. Garnish with scallions and sesame seeds and serve immediately.

Per Serving: Calories: 405; Fat: 4g; Carbohydrates: 79g; Fiber: 8g; Sugar: 10g; Protein: 13g; Sodium: 1,865mg

Lemon Mushroom Orzo with Spinach and Peas

SERVES 6   **PREP TIME:** 10 MINUTES   **COOK TIME:** 15 MINUTES
NUT-FREE, SOY-FREE

Orzo is a short-cut pasta shaped like rice that is a fabulous alternative to heavy, large pastas like penne or fusilli. Orzo can be boiled and drained like regular pasta, or it can be low-simmered like arborio rice for a rich, creamy risotto-like consistency. In this recipe, we'll treat the orzo like pasta and whip up a fabulous veg-loaded dish that is delicious served hot or cold. If fresh peas aren't in season, use frozen instead.

4 cups low-sodium vegetable broth or water

1½ cups uncooked orzo

1½ cups fresh or frozen green peas

1 tablespoon grapeseed oil or extra-virgin olive oil

1 small yellow onion, diced

1 (8-ounce) package cremini or button mushrooms, stemmed, caps sliced

2 cups packed baby spinach

1 teaspoon grated lemon zest

3 teaspoons lemon juice

½ teaspoon kosher salt

½ teaspoon freshly ground black pepper

1. In a large pot, bring the vegetable broth to a boil over high heat. Stir in the orzo and cook until al dente, 8 to 10 minutes. During the last 2 minutes of cooking, add the peas. Drain and transfer to a large bowl.

2. Meanwhile, in a large skillet, heat the oil over medium-high heat until it shimmers. Add the onion and mushrooms and cook until the onions are soft and the mushrooms are golden, about 5 minutes. Add the spinach and cook, stirring constantly, until the spinach is wilted, about 2 minutes.

3. Add the cooked vegetables to the orzo bowl, along with the lemon zest, lemon juice, salt, and pepper, and toss well to combine before serving.

Cooking Tip: You can serve this warm, or chill in the refrigerator for a minimum of 1 hour and serve as a cold orzo salad.

Per Serving: Calories: 240; Fat: 3g; Carbohydrates: 43g; Fiber: 9g; Sugar: 6g; Protein: 10g; Sodium: 250mg

sta e Ceci (Italian-Style nickpea and Pasta Stew)

SERVES 6   **PREP TIME:** 5 MINUTES   **COOK TIME:** 15 MINUTES
ONE-POT, FREEZER-FRIENDLY, NUT-FREE, SOY-FREE

Pasta e ceci (or "pasta and chickpeas") is a rich, comforting, low-fuss meal made with ditalini (very short tubes) or another small pasta and chickpeas, which is flavored with garlic, rosemary, and tomato. And, if you're me, a little bit of heat, too.

2 tablespoons grapeseed or extra-virgin olive oil

2 teaspoons jarred minced garlic or 4 garlic cloves, minced

2 whole rosemary sprigs

½ teaspoon crushed red pepper flakes

3 tablespoons tomato paste

2 (15-ounce) cans no-salt-added chickpeas, drained and rinsed, divided

5 cups low-sodium vegetable broth, divided

8 ounces uncooked ditalini or elbow macaroni

2 cups baby spinach or chopped baby kale

¼ cup nutritional yeast

½ teaspoon onion powder

½ teaspoon kosher salt

½ teaspoon freshly ground black pepper

1. In a large stockpot or Dutch oven, heat the oil over medium-high heat, then add the garlic, rosemary, red pepper flakes, and tomato paste. Cook, stirring frequently, until fragrant, about 4 minutes. Remove and discard the rosemary sprigs.

2. Add 1 can of chickpeas and 2 cups of vegetable broth and, using a potato masher or a fork, mash the chickpeas slightly. Then add the remaining can of chickpeas and 3 cups of vegetable broth and bring to a boil.

3. Add the pasta, reduce the heat to a simmer, and cook for 1 minute less than the package directions, stirring frequently, until the liquid has reduced to between a sauce and a soup.

4. Remove from the heat and add the spinach, nutritional yeast, onion powder, salt, and black pepper and stir, letting the residual heat wilt the spinach. Serve.

Cooking Tip: Like most soups and stews, this dish is a great freezer meal. To make this ahead and freeze, stop the cooking process after the pasta is done, allow it to cool to room temperature, then divide it into freezer-safe containers or resealable bags. To reheat, thaw in the refrigerator overnight, then gently warm in a pot, adding extra water or broth to loosen if needed. Once it's hot, stir in the baby spinach, nutritional yeast, salt, and pepper.

Per Serving: Calories: 345; Fat: 8g; Carbohydrates: 54g; Fiber: 9g; Sugar: 6g; Protein: 15g; Sodium: 409mg

Sun-Dried Tomato and Roasted Red Pepper Fettuccine Alfredo

SERVES 5   PREP TIME: 10 MINUTES   **COOK TIME:** 15 MINUTES
NUT-FREE, OIL-FREE, SOY-FREE

The salty, briny, and sweet combination of sun-dried tomatoes and roasted red peppers makes for the perfect twist on fettuccine alfredo. Coconut milk replaces the heavy cream in this sauce to keep it dairy-free. Regular coconut milk will yield a creamier, richer sauce, but it does have more fat, so consider using a light coconut milk to keep this dish lower in fat.

8 ounces uncooked whole-wheat fettuccine

3 teaspoons jarred minced garlic

½ cup chopped jarred sun-dried tomatoes

½ cup chopped roasted red peppers

½ teaspoon crushed red pepper flakes

1 (14-ounce) can artichoke hearts packed in water, drained

1 tablespoon water, plus more if needed

2 cups packed baby spinach

1 (14-ounce) can regular or light coconut milk

3 tablespoons chopped fresh basil

1. Bring a large pot of water to a boil over high heat and cook the fettuccine according to the package directions. Drain and set aside.

2. Meanwhile, heat a large skillet over medium heat. Combine the garlic, sun-dried tomatoes, roasted red peppers, red pepper flakes, and artichoke hearts and cook, stirring constantly, for 3 to 4 minutes, or until the garlic and tomatoes are fragrant. If the skillet starts to get dry, add a tablespoon or two of water. Add the baby spinach and stir constantly until wilted, about 2 minutes.

3. Add the coconut milk and simmer until the sauce is thick enough to coat the back of a spoon, about 5 minutes. Add the drained pasta to the skillet, tossing to coat the noodles in the sauce. Top with fresh basil before serving.

Cooking Tip: Because the garlic and sun-dried tomatoes (and possibly the roasted red peppers) are packed in oil, we're not adding any extra to the skillet—so don't pat the tomatoes or peppers dry before adding them to the skillet. To keep the skillet from getting dry or to avoid burning the garlic, keep the temperature lower (medium heat only) and add a tablespoon or two of water as needed.

Per Serving: Calories: 354; Fat: 17g; Carbohydrates: 49g; Fiber: 12g; Sugar: 7g; Protein: 10g; Sodium: 305mg

Creamy Pumpkin Penne

SERVES 5   **PREP TIME:** 10 MINUTES   **COOK TIME:** 15 MINUTES
NUT-FREE, OIL-FREE, SOY-FREE

I always think of autumn when I make this pasta because of its bright orange color and warm fall flavors. Pumpkin pie spice is a blend of cinnamon, nutmeg, ginger, and cloves and is available in almost every grocery store. It's an economical and time-saving way to add all those warm fall spices to a dish without having to measure them out. Plus, it takes up less space in your pantry.

1 (16-ounce) box uncooked whole-wheat penne

1 (10-ounce) bag frozen diced butternut squash

2 tablespoons low-sodium vegetable broth or water, plus more as needed

½ medium yellow onion, diced

1 teaspoon jarred minced garlic, or 2 garlic cloves, minced

1½ cups regular or light coconut milk

1 (15-ounce) can plain pumpkin

¼ teaspoon crushed red pepper flakes

½ teaspoon pumpkin pie spice

½ cup nutritional yeast

2 cups packed baby spinach

1. Bring a large pot of water to a boil over high heat and cook the pasta according to the package directions. During the last 2 minutes of cooking, add the squash. Drain and set aside.

2. Meanwhile, in a large skillet heat the broth over medium heat. When it's just starting to simmer, add the onion and garlic and cook, stirring constantly, for 5 minutes, or until the onion starts to soften. Add more broth or water if needed, 1 teaspoon at a time, to keep the skillet from drying out.

3. Add the coconut milk, pumpkin, red pepper flakes, pumpkin pie spice, and nutritional yeast and stir to combine into a pumpkin-colored sauce. Simmer for 10 minutes, or until the sauce thickens slightly.

4. Add the cooked pasta and baby spinach to the skillet, tossing to coat and to wilt the spinach. Remove from the heat and serve.

Per Serving: Calories: 559; Fat: 16g; Carbohydrates: 89g; Fiber: 15g; Sugar: 11g; Protein: 22g; Sodium: 34mg

Linguini with Artichokes in Lemon Dill Sauce

SERVES 5 **PREP TIME:** 10 MINUTES **COOK TIME:** 15 MINUTES
NUT-FREE, SOY-FREE

In my pre-vegan days, fish cooked in a lemon dill sauce was always a favorite. I created this dish to enjoy a similar flavor profile without the fish. Because artichokes are brined, they help give the sauce a similar salty, ocean flavor. If I'm looking to make this dish even more substantial, I'll bake some vegan fishless fillets and add them to the skillet just before serving.

1 (16-ounce) package uncooked
    whole-wheat linguini
1 tablespoon grapeseed oil or extra-virgin
    olive oil
½ medium yellow onion, finely diced
1 (14-ounce) can artichoke hearts packed
    in water, drained
1 tablespoon lemon zest
½ teaspoon jarred minced garlic, or 1 garlic
    clove, minced

2 tablespoons lemon juice
½ cup low-sodium vegetable broth
1 (15-ounce) can full-fat coconut milk
1 tablespoon nutritional yeast
2 tablespoons chopped fresh dill, or
    1 tablespoon dried dill
½ teaspoon kosher salt
½ teaspoon freshly ground black pepper
1 teaspoon cornstarch mixed with
    2 teaspoons cold water

1. Bring a large pot of water to a boil over high heat and cook the pasta according to the package directions. Drain and set aside.

2. Meanwhile, in a large skillet, heat the oil over medium-high heat. Add the onion, artichokes, and lemon zest and cook until the onions are translucent, about 5 minutes. Add the garlic and lemon juice and cook, stirring constantly, for 30 seconds.

3. Add the broth, coconut milk, nutritional yeast, dill, salt, and pepper and bring to just under a boil. Reduce the heat to medium-low and simmer for 10 minutes.

4. Add the cornstarch mixture and cook, stirring constantly, for 2 minutes. Remove from the heat and add the cooked linguini to the sauce, tossing to coat. Enjoy.

Per Serving: Calories: 529; Fat: 20g; Carbohydrates: 81g; Fiber: 15g; Sugar: 6g; Protein: 17g; Sodium: 344mg

Fusilli with Butter Chicken Sauce and Cherry Tomatoes

SERVES 5   **PREP TIME:** 10 MINUTES   **COOK TIME:** 20 MINUTES
NUT-FREE, SOY-FREE

Butter chicken sauce is a classic Indian flavor combination that works surprisingly well with pasta. Despite its name, it contains neither butter nor chicken, and with a simple modification, this traditionally vegetarian sauce becomes a part of a delicious vegan meal. If you're looking to add more protein, you could stir in some chickpeas and spinach, or panfry some extra-firm tofu cubes.

1 (16-ounce) box uncooked whole-wheat fusilli

1 tablespoon grapeseed oil or extra-virgin olive oil

1 medium yellow onion, diced

1 (14-ounce) can cherry tomatoes, drained, or 1 pint fresh cherry tomatoes

1 teaspoon jarred minced garlic or 2 garlic cloves, minced

1 tablespoon jarred minced ginger, or 1 thumb-size piece fresh ginger, grated

1 tablespoon ground cumin

1 teaspoon mild curry powder

¼ to ½ teaspoon ground cayenne pepper

½ teaspoon kosher salt

¼ cup plus 2 tablespoons no-salt-added tomato paste

1 (14-ounce) can light coconut milk

1. Bring a large pot of water to a boil over high heat and cook the pasta according to the package directions. Drain and set aside.

2. Meanwhile, in a large skillet, heat the oil over medium-high heat until it shimmers. Add the onion and tomatoes and cook for 3 to 4 minutes, or until the onions are translucent and the tomatoes soften.

3. Add the garlic and ginger and cook, stirring constantly, for 30 seconds, then add the cumin, curry powder, cayenne pepper, salt, tomato paste, and coconut milk. Stir to combine. Simmer for 10 minutes, until sauce bubbles and thickens slightly.

4. Add the pasta to the saucepan, tossing well to coat before serving.

Per Serving: Calories: 446; Fat: 11g; Carbohydrates: 79g; Fiber: 11g; Sugar: 8g; Protein: 15g; Sodium: 235mg

15-Minute White Mac and "Cheese" with Broccoli

SERVES 4   PREP TIME: 5 MINUTES   **COOK TIME:** 10 MINUTES
NUT-FREE, OIL-FREE

A good mac and cheese should be rich, creamy, and velvety smooth. My 15-minute version checks all those boxes—and it's super fast, too. My trick is cannellini beans, which are blended with plant-based milk and seasonings to create a delicious sauce. This version is oil-free, but if you're amenable to a little bit of oil in your diet, I recommend adding 1 or 2 teaspoons of good extra-virgin olive oil while blending to add smoothness and flavor. If you prefer a classic orange mac and cheese sauce, add ⅛ teaspoon of turmeric and ¼ teaspoon of paprika to the sauce while blending.

8 ounces uncooked small shells or elbow
  macaroni

1 cup broccoli florets

1 cup no-salt-added cannellini beans,
  drained and rinsed

½ cup unsweetened plain soy milk

5 tablespoons nutritional yeast

½ teaspoon kosher salt

⅛ teaspoon garlic powder

⅛ teaspoon onion powder

½ teaspoon apple cider vinegar

1. Bring a large pot of water to a boil over high heat and cook the pasta according to the package directions. Add the broccoli during the last 2 minutes of cooking. Drain and return to the pot. Set aside.

2. Meanwhile, in a blender or food processor, process the beans, soy milk, nutritional yeast, salt, garlic powder, onion powder, and vinegar until smooth.

3. Pour the sauce over the cooked pasta and broccoli and stir to combine, letting the residual heat from the pasta warm the sauce. Serve warm.

Variation Tip: Nutritional yeast adds a rich nutty and cheesy flavor to this sauce, but if you want a more authentic "cheese" flavor, you could swap it for ⅓ cup of your favorite vegan shreds, like Daiya Farmhouse Block, in Cheddar or Monterey Jack flavor. You'll need to warm the sauce over low heat for 5 minutes while you stir in the shreds to ensure they melt evenly into the sauce. This can be done while the pasta is cooking.

Per Serving: Calories: 316; Fat: 2g; Carbohydrates: 56g; Fiber: 8g; Sugar: 2g; Protein: 17g; Sodium: 181mg

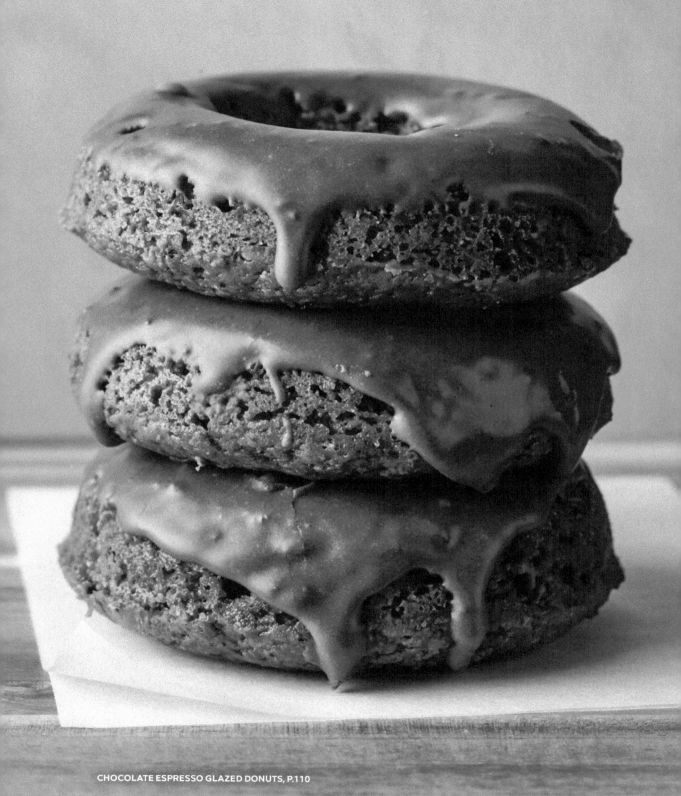

CHOCOLATE ESPRESSO GLAZED DONUTS, P.110

Desserts

Coconut Macaroons   104

Carrot Cake Energy Bites   105

Bakery-Style Giant Chocolate Chip Cookies   106

Whipped Shortbread Cookies   108

Maple Chocolate Hazelnut Mousse   109

Chocolate Espresso Glazed Donuts   110

Grapefruit, Lime, and Mint Yogurt Parfait   112

Apricot Peach Crisp   113

Bananas Foster Sundaes   114

Cherry Cheesecake Jars   115

Coconut Macaroons

MAKES 24 COOKIES   **PREP TIME:** 10 MINUTES   **COOK TIME:** 20 MINUTES
GLUTEN-FREE, OIL-FREE, SOY-FREE

This is my favorite old-school macaroon recipe. Unlike the French macaron, which is made from almond flour and egg whites, macaroons (note the extra O) are delicious little mounds of shredded coconut and egg whites. For obvious reasons, I'm using coconut milk instead of egg, which not only binds the macaroons but also adds more delicious coconut flavor. You can dip or drizzle your macaroons with chocolate, or add unsweetened cocoa powder to make them fully chocolate.

3 cups unsweetened
   shredded coconut
1 cup canned light coconut milk
⅓ cup pure maple syrup
⅓ cup gluten-free flour blend

2 teaspoons pure vanilla extract
⅛ teaspoon kosher salt
⅓ cup slivered or chopped almonds
   (optional)

1. Preheat the oven to 350°F. Line a large baking sheet with parchment paper.

2. In a large bowl, combine the shredded coconut, coconut milk, maple syrup, flour, vanilla, salt, and almonds (if using) and mix well.

3. Use a 2-tablespoon ice-cream scoop to scoop out even, well-packed scoops of dough, and place them on the prepared baking sheet about 1 inch apart. Bake for 20 minutes, or until just golden.

4. Let cool completely before enjoying.

Cooking Tip: To make these next-level macaroons, melt ½ cup of dark chocolate chips in the microwave in 30-second intervals (to a maximum of 90 seconds) until smooth. Transfer to a shallow bowl and dip the bottoms of the macaroons in the chocolate and then in colorful sprinkles before setting them down to dry. Store in an airtight container in the refrigerator for up to 5 days.

Per Serving (2 cookies): Calories: 90; Fat: 7g; Carbohydrates: 7g; Fiber: 2g; Sugar: 3g; Protein: 1g; Sodium: 11mg

Carrot Cake Energy Bites

MAKES 12 BITES   PREP TIME: 30 MINUTES
ONE-POT, GLUTEN-FREE, NUT-FREE, OIL-FREE, SOY-FREE

I have a carrot cake–loving family. My brother, husband, and eldest daughter all list carrot cake as their favorite of all cakes. They also happen to be gluten- and sugar-sensitive, so I created these delish little energy bites to mimic all the classic flavors of carrot cake, without the gluten or refined sugar.

½ cup shredded coconut

3 Medjool dates, pitted

4 dried apricots

2 tablespoons unsweetened applesauce

2 tablespoons pure maple syrup

1 teaspoon pure vanilla extract

¼ cup coconut flour

1 cup gluten-free oats

½ teaspoon pumpkin pie spice

1 cup shredded carrots

1. Line a tray or a large plate with parchment paper. Put the shredded coconut on a shallow plate.

2. In a food processor fitted with an S blade or a small electric food chopper, combine the dates, apricots, applesauce, maple syrup, and vanilla. Pulse until combined and the dates and apricots are broken down into small pieces. Add the coconut flour, oats, pumpkin pie spice, and carrots and pulse until a sticky dough forms.

3. Scoop out a tablespoon at a time, roll into a ball, and place on the lined tray. When all the dough is rolled out, toss each ball in the shredded coconut before returning it to the tray.

4. Chill for 10 to 15 minutes before eating. Store the energy bites in an airtight container in the refrigerator for up to 4 days.

Variation Tip: If carrot cake isn't your thing, try key lime pie energy bites instead. In a food processor, combine 2 cups of unsweetened shredded coconut, ½ cup of gluten-free oats, 2 tablespoons of pure maple syrup or agave, 2 tablespoons of melted coconut oil, 1 teaspoon of pure vanilla extract, and the zest of 8 key limes. Process until a sticky dough forms, roll out into 1-inch balls, and toss in more shredded coconut to coat.

Per Serving (1 bite): Calories: 91; Fat: 3g; Carbohydrates: 15g; Fiber: 3g; Sugar: 8g; Protein: 2g; Sodium: 14mg

Bakery-Style Giant Chocolate Chip Cookies

MAKES 15 COOKIES   **PREP TIME:** 10 MINUTES   **COOK TIME:** 12 MINUTES
NUT-FREE, SOY-FREE

I firmly believe you cannot be miserable when eating a cookie. And trust me, I've tested that theory plenty. These are one of my all-time favorite cookies and are always a crowd-pleaser. They're modeled after a famous New York City bakery that is known for making these giant cake-like cookies. To make my version slightly healthier, I've replaced some of the refined sugar with natural unsweetened applesauce.

1¼ cups all-purpose flour

¾ cup cake flour

1 teaspoon cornstarch

½ teaspoon baking powder

½ teaspoon baking soda

½ teaspoon kosher salt

½ cup vegan butter, cold

½ cup packed light brown sugar

¼ cup granulated sugar

¼ cup plus 2 tablespoons unsweetened
   applesauce

1 cup dairy-free mini chocolate chips

1. Preheat the oven to 400°F. Line three baking sheets with parchment paper.

2. In a large bowl, sift together the all-purpose and cake flours, cornstarch, baking powder, baking soda, and salt. Set aside.

3. In another large bowl, using a hand mixer (or in a stand mixer fitted with the paddle attachment), cream the butter for 30 seconds on medium-high speed. Add the brown sugar and cream until fully incorporated, about 1 minute, scraping down the sides as necessary. Repeat with the granulated sugar. Add the apple-sauce and mix until it's just incorporated.

4. Reduce the speed to slow and gradually add the flour mixture, about ⅓ cup at a time. Mix until just combined and no flour streaks are left. Using a rubber spatula, gently fold in the chocolate chips.

5. Using a 2-inch ice-cream scoop, drop scoopfuls of dough on the prepared baking sheets, putting no more than six cookies on each sheet. Bake for 10 to 12 minutes, or until the tops are golden but the cookies look slightly underdone or soft (they will continue to cook as they rest on the baking sheet).

6. Let the cookies rest on the baking sheet for 15 minutes before transferring to a wire rack to cool completely. Enjoy.

Ingredient Tip: Cake flour is a lighter, lower-gluten flour that is often used in cakes and cupcakes to give them a lighter, fluffier texture. If you don't have cake flour at home, you can easily make it by measuring 1 cup of all-purpose flour, then removing 2 tablespoons and replacing it with 2 tablespoons of cornstarch and whisking well to combine.

Per Serving (1 cookie): Calories: 242; Fat: 11g; Carbohydrates: 34g; Fiber: 2g; Sugar: 18g; Protein: 3g; Sodium: 152mg

Whipped Shortbread Cookies

MAKES 4 DOZEN COOKIES   **PREP TIME:** 10 MINUTES   **COOK TIME:** 20 MINUTES
NUT-FREE, SOY-FREE

Admittedly, these are a once-in-a-while cookie treat. I usually make them around the holidays to share at a potluck or as a homemade gift in a fancy tin. They are delicious shortbread meltaway bites that are as fun to make as they are to eat but offer little in the "healthy" department. I've adapted my original recipe to use light spelt flour, which is healthier than all-purpose wheat flour and doesn't change the light and airy consistency of the cookie too much.

1½ cups vegan butter, softened

¾ cup confectioners' sugar

½ teaspoon pure vanilla or almond extract

2¼ cups light spelt flour

¾ cups cornstarch

2 tablespoons vegan sprinkles

1. Preheat the oven to 300°F. Line two large baking sheets with parchment paper.

2. In a large bowl, using an electric hand mixer, cream the butter, confectioners' sugar, and vanilla until light and fluffy, at least 5 minutes. (This could also be done in a stand mixer fitted with the paddle attachment.) Gradually add the flour and cornstarch, beating until well blended.

3. Using a melon baller or a teaspoon, scoop out balls of dough, rolling them between your hands to form little balls about 1 inch in diameter. Place on the prepared baking sheets and press each ball with a lightly floured fork.

4. Top with sprinkles and bake for 18 to 20 minutes, or until the bottoms are lightly browned. Cool completely before enjoying. Store any leftovers in an airtight container at room temperature for up to 4 days.

Per Serving (2 cookies): Calories: 176; Fat: 11g; Carbohydrates: 17g; Fiber: 2g; Sugar: 4g; Protein: 2g; Sodium: 105mg

Maple Chocolate Hazelnut Mousse

SERVES 4 PREP TIME: 20 MINUTES **COOK TIME:** 10 MINUTES
GLUTEN-FREE

Chocolate mousse may seem complicated, but I promise you, it's really easy to make and is a fantastic treat any day of the week. For a smooth, whipped consistency similar to mousse made from egg whites, I recommend using silken tofu. However, if you want to avoid soy, substitute 1 large or 2 small ripe avocados instead. You won't taste the avocado, but you will get a smooth, pudding-like dessert.

½ cup raw hazelnuts

½ cup, pure maple syrup, plus 2 tablespoons

1 (4-ounce) bar dark chocolate
   (70 percent cocoa)

1 teaspoon coconut oil

1 (12-ounce) package silken tofu

2 tablespoons unsweetened cocoa powder

½ teaspoon pure vanilla extract

¼ teaspoon kosher salt

1.   Line a small baking sheet with wax paper or parchment paper.

2.   In a small saucepan over high heat, combine the hazelnuts and ½ cup of maple syrup and cook for 3 to 5 minutes, or until the nuts are golden brown and fragrant. Transfer to the prepared baking sheet and chill in the refrigerator while you make the mousse.

3.   In a microwave-safe bowl, combine the chocolate and oil and microwave in 30-second intervals (to a maximum of 90 seconds) until smooth. Transfer to a blender or food processor and add the tofu, cocoa powder, remaining 2 tablespoons of maple syrup, the vanilla, and salt. Process until smooth. Spoon into four dessert cups, parfait dishes, mason jars, or bowls and chill in the freezer for 15 to 20 minutes.

4.   Meanwhile, chop the hazelnuts. Remove the chilled mousse from the freezer and top with chopped maple hazelnuts before enjoying.

Per Serving: Calories: 456; Fat: 26g; Carbohydrates: 52g; Fiber: 6g; Sugar: 37g; Protein: 9g; Sodium: 97mg

Chocolate Espresso Glazed Donuts

SERVES 6 **PREP TIME:** 10 MINUTES **COOK TIME:** 12 MINUTES
SOY-FREE

These baked cake-like donuts are deliciously rich treats that require simple ingredients and come together in just minutes. I make mine in a donut pan, but if you don't have one, use a standard muffin tin with rolled-up little balls of aluminum foil in the center to form the hole, or bake them like cupcakes and cut out the hole once they cool. (You'll have to increase your baking time a little for this method.)

FOR THE DONUTS

3 tablespoons vegan butter, melted, plus
   more for greasing

1 cup all-purpose flour

¼ cup unsweetened dark cocoa powder

1 teaspoon baking powder

½ cup granulated sugar

1 teaspoon espresso powder or instant
   coffee granules

¼ teaspoon kosher salt

FOR THE GLAZE

¾ cup plain unsweetened almond milk

1 teaspoon pure vanilla extract

1 cup confectioners' sugar

¼ cup Dutch-process dark cocoa powder

½ teaspoon pure vanilla extract

4 to 5 tablespoons plain unsweetened
   almond milk

1. Preheat the oven to 350°F. Grease a 6-hole donut pan with vegan butter.

2. In a large bowl, sift together the flour, cocoa powder, and baking powder. Then add the sugar, espresso powder, and salt and whisk to combine. Make a well in the center of the bowl and add the almond milk, vegan butter, and vanilla. Mix until just combined and no flour streaks are left in the batter.

3. Spoon or pipe the batter into the prepared donut pan, filling each cavity about three-quarters full. Bake for 10 to 12 minutes, or until a cake tester or a toothpick inserted in the donut comes out clean. Cool in the pan for 5 minutes, then transfer to a wire rack set on top of a parchment-lined baking sheet to cool.

4. Meanwhile, make the glaze. In a small bowl, combine the confectioners' sugar, cocoa powder, vanilla, and 4 tablespoons of almond milk and whisk until smooth. If the glaze is too thick, add the remaining 1 tablespoon of milk and whisk until it's smooth and pourable. Spoon the glaze onto the cooling donuts and enjoy.

Variation Tip: Try swapping the vegan butter for the same amount of melted coconut oil to make this dessert less processed. Virgin coconut oil is made from the fresh milk of a coconut and is cold-pressed, preserving most of the antioxidants and other nutritional benefits of coconut. It has a low smoke point, so it's not great for panfrying but works well in baked goods.

Per Serving (1 donut): Calories: 300; Fat: 7g; Carbohydrates: 57g; Fiber: 3g; Sugar: 37g; Protein: 4g; Sodium: 212mg

Grapefruit, Lime, and Mint Yogurt Parfait

SERVES 6   PREP TIME: 30 MINUTES
ONE-POT, GLUTEN-FREE, OIL-FREE, SOY-FREE

Grapefruit-lime yogurt parfaits are a lovely light and tart dessert, or a great breakfast idea, too. I love using fresh red grapefruits, as they are naturally sweeter than pink- or white-fleshed ones. If you can't find fresh, or you want to make this dessert even faster, you can use sliced fresh grapefruit packed in light syrup and gently rinsed. Try to avoid using "packed in water" versions, as they are generally artificially sweetened with sucralose or aspartame.

4 cups plain unsweetened coconut yogurt

2 teaspoons grated lime zest

2 tablespoons lime juice

4 large ruby red grapefruits

2 tablespoons pure maple syrup, divided

½ cup roasted, unsalted pecans, roughly chopped, divided

1. In a large bowl, mix the yogurt, lime zest, and lime juice. Set aside.

2. Cut the grapefruits into segments by cutting off the tops and bottoms so that the grapefruits can stand upright on a cutting board. Use your knife to cut away the grapefruit rind and then cut in between the white parts to remove the fruit.

3. Divide half of the grapefruit segments among six dessert glasses, and top with half of the yogurt. Repeat with another layer each of grapefruit and yogurt, then drizzle each parfait with a teaspoon of maple syrup and about 1 tablespoon of chopped pecans. Enjoy immediately.

Variation Tip: Swap this light and summery recipe for the classic fall flavors of an apple pie parfait. Start with 2 cups of your favorite low-sugar granola (I like Go Raw Super-Simple Sprouted Granola) and divide 1 cup of it among 4 dessert glasses. Add ⅓ cup of vanilla coconut yogurt to each glass. In a small bowl, combine 1 cup of unsweetened applesauce, ½ teaspoon of ground cinnamon, and ¼ teaspoon of ground nutmeg, then divide that evenly among the four glasses. Top each with another ¼ cup of granola.

Per Serving: Calories: 247; Fat: 12g; Carbohydrates: 37g; Fiber: 6g; Sugar: 20g; Protein: 3g; Sodium: 31mg

Apricot Peach Crisp

SERVES 6 TO 8   PREP TIME: 10 MINUTES   **COOK TIME:** 15 MINUTES
FREEZER-FRIENDLY, NUT-FREE, SOY-FREE

Fruit crisps are my secret weapon when I want to serve a pie dessert but don't want the hassle of actually making a pie. Fruit crisps are easy to assemble and bake up in 15 to 20 minutes, making them a perfect weeknight dessert. I'm using tart, tangy apricots and sweet, juicy peaches in this recipe, but any combination of fresh, canned, or frozen fruit works, like mixed berries, apple and cinnamon, or a mix of stone fruits and berries.

10 fresh apricots, halved

2 (10-ounce) bags frozen sliced peaches

4 tablespoons coconut sugar, divided

½ teaspoon ground ginger

¼ teaspoon ground cinnamon

¼ cups quick-cooking oats

2 tablespoons shredded unsweetened coconut

¼ cup all-purpose flour or light spelt flour

3 tablespoons virgin coconut oil, solid

1. Preheat the oven to 400°F.

2. In a 9-by-13-inch baking dish, combine the apricots, peaches, 2 tablespoons of sugar, the ginger, and cinnamon. Toss to coat and spread in an even layer.

3. In a small bowl, combine the oats, the remaining 2 tablespoons of sugar, the shredded coconut, flour, and oil and mash until mixed. Sprinkle over the top of the fruit. Bake for 15 minutes, or until bubbly. Serve.

Cooking Tip: Fruit crisps freeze beautifully, making them a great make-ahead dessert. To freeze a fruit crisp, assemble the dish in an aluminum foil casserole dish, wrap in plastic wrap, then place in an airtight container or freezer-safe bag and store for up to 4 months. Thaw overnight in the refrigerator, then bake at 350°F until bubbly and warmed through. You can also freeze a baked crisp—just let it cool completely before freezing.

Per Serving: Calories: 185; Fat: 8g; Carbohydrates: 27g; Fiber: 3g; Sugar: 18g; Protein: 2g; Sodium: 18mg

Bananas Foster Sundaes

SERVES 4 **PREP TIME:** 10 MINUTES **COOK TIME:** 5 MINUTES
ONE-POT, GLUTEN-FREE, SOY-FREE

Bananas foster is an elegant, flamboyant (and flammable) restaurant dessert in which bananas are cooked tableside in butter, cinnamon, and sugar, then ignited with rum and banana liqueur to produce flames, and served over vanilla ice cream. But if you prefer your dessert without theatrics, this at-home, alcohol-free version works just as well. I'm swapping the rum for almond extract and adding the zest and juice of an orange to give this dessert a bit of punch.

1 tablespoon vegan butter

3 tablespoons coconut sugar

½ teaspoon ground cinnamon

¼ teaspoon ground nutmeg

1 teaspoon orange zest

1 tablespoon freshly squeezed orange juice

3 large, firm bananas, cut into 1-inch-slices

2 tablespoons chopped roasted pecans

¼ teaspoon almond extract

2 cups (1 pint) dairy-free vanilla ice cream, divided

1. In a large skillet melt the butter over medium-low heat. Swirl until melted. Stir in the sugar, cinnamon, nutmeg, orange zest, and orange juice, then add the bananas, pecans, and vanilla, stirring gently to coat. Cook for 3 minutes, or until the bananas are just softened and glazed. Remove from the heat.

2. Add ½ cup of ice cream to a sundae dish and top with ¼ of the banana mixture. Repeat with the remaining three dishes. Serve immediately.

Per Serving: Calories: 298; Fat: 13g; Carbohydrates: 53g; Fiber: 8g; Sugar: 30g; Protein: 2g; Sodium: 78mg

Cherry Cheesecake Jars

MAKES 12 JARS   PREP TIME: 30 MINUTES
NUT-FREE, SOY-FREE

What's better than a slice of cherry cheesecake? Your very own jar that you don't have to share! These little mason jar cheesecakes are the perfect no-bake treat when you just want a little taste of something sweet. To keep this dessert down to 30 minutes, I'm using store-bought vegan cream cheese, but if you have time to spare, you could use soaked, blended cashews. Condensed coconut milk replaces sugar, and cherry pie filling is a quick alternative to stovetop cooked fruit. I like to use Lotus Biscoff cookies for the crust and Daiya cream cheese in this recipe.

12 vegan graham crackers or gingersnap cookies

¼ cup virgin coconut oil, melted

1 (8-ounce) container dairy-free cream cheese

1 (11-ounce) can condensed coconut milk

⅓ cup lemon juice

1 teaspoon pure vanilla extract

1 (21-ounce) can cherry pie filling

1. Place the graham crackers in a resealable bag and crush using a rolling pin or your hands until they're finely ground. Transfer to a bowl and mix with the oil. Divide evenly and press into 12 small mason jars.

2. In a large bowl, using an electric hand mixer, beat the cream cheese until fluffy, about 4 minutes. Gradually beat in the coconut milk, then gently stir in the lemon juice and vanilla.

3. Divide the cream cheese mixture evenly among the mason jars, then top with a layer of cherry pie filling. Serve immediately or seal each jar and store in the refrigerator for up to 4 days.

Per Serving (1 jar): Calories: 298; Fat: 14g; Carbohydrates: 40g; Fiber: <1g; Sugar: 19g; Protein: 2g; Sodium: 183mg

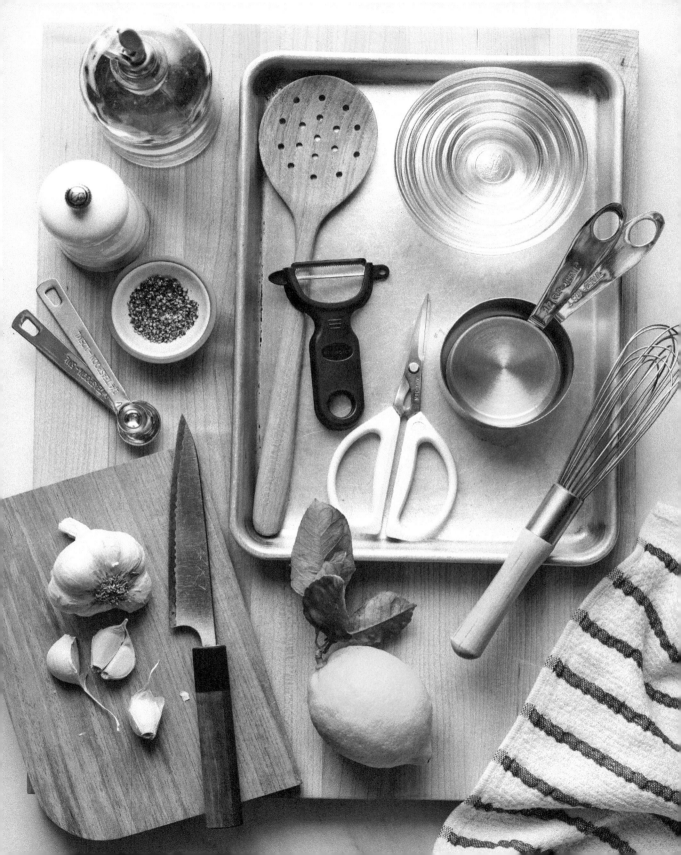

MEASUREMENT CONVERSIONS

VOLUME EQUIVALENTS	U.S. STANDARD	U.S. STANDARD (OUNCES)	METRIC (APPROXIMATE)
LIQUID	2 tablespoons	1 fl. oz.	30 mL
	¼ cup	2 fl. oz.	60 mL
	½ cup	4 fl. oz.	120 mL
	1 cup	8 fl. oz.	240 mL
	1½ cups	12 fl. oz.	355 mL
	2 cups or 1 pint	16 fl. oz.	475 mL
	4 cups or 1 quart	32 fl. oz.	1 L
	1 gallon	128 fl. oz.	4 L
DRY	⅛ teaspoon	–	0.5 mL
	¼ teaspoon	–	1 mL
	½ teaspoon	–	2 mL
	¾ teaspoon	–	4 mL
	1 teaspoon	–	5 mL
	1 tablespoon	–	15 mL
	¼ cup	–	59 mL
	⅓ cup	–	79 mL
	½ cup	–	118 mL
	⅔ cup	–	156 mL
	¾ cup	–	177 mL
	1 cup	–	235 mL
	2 cups or 1 pint	–	475 mL
	3 cups	–	700 mL
	4 cups or 1 quart	–	1 L
	½ gallon	–	2 L
	1 gallon	–	4 L

OVEN TEMPERATURES

FAHRENHEIT	CELSIUS (APPROXIMATE)
250°F	120°C
300°F	150°C
325°F	165°C
350°F	180°C
375°F	190°C
400°F	200°C
425°F	220°C
450°F	230°C

WEIGHT EQUIVALENTS

U.S. STANDARD	METRIC (APPROXIMATE)
½ ounce	15 g
1 ounce	30 g
2 ounces	60 g
4 ounces	115 g
8 ounces	225 g
12 ounces	340 g
16 ounces or 1 pound	455 g

RESOURCES

Websites

Forks Over Knives
ForksOverKnives.com

This is the companion website to the groundbreaking 2011 documentary *Forks Over Knives*, which illustrates the connection between a healthy plant-based diet and overall well-being. This website contains numerous plant-based recipes, meal plans, and nutritional information.

NutritionFacts.org
NutritionFacts.org

This is a great resource for those who want to learn more about the science behind plant-based eating. Dr. Michael Greger has posted more than a thousand bite-size, easily digestible videos here that analyze the latest developments in nutritional research.

One Green Planet
OneGreenPlanet.org

One Green Planet is an online guide to making conscious and compassionate choices that help people, animals, and the planet. This website contains numerous plant-based recipes and health information, as well as articles on a wide variety of topics.

VegNews
VegNews.com

VegNews is a popular magazine about all things vegan: recipes, travel, product and restaurant reviews, news, lifestyle, and more. Their website provides lots of articles and resources covering a wide range of vegan topics.

SHOPPING

Amazon

Amazon.com

Amazon is a huge online destination for kitchen equipment and tools, plus many specialty vegan and international food ingredients. Amazon has various subscription programs that may save you money if there are things you buy often from them.

Target

Target.com

Target sells a wide variety of kitchen equipment and tools both in their physical stores and online. They also carry a decent number of plant-based ingredients.

Trader Joe's

TraderJoes.com

Trader Joe's is a great resource for plant-based ingredients and products. They do carry a lot of convenience foods, but they have plenty of whole foods, too, as well as great produce and a good selection of frozen fruits, vegetables, and cooked whole grains.

Whole Foods

WholeFoodsMarket.com

Whole Foods is a national grocery chain that offers organic and plant-based groceries, along with produce and other health-related products.

INDEX

A

Almond Ricotta Toasts, Tomato and, 21
Apricot Peach Crisp, 113
Artichokes
  Lemon Quinoa Artichoke Salad, 49
  Linguini with Artichokes in Lemon Dill Sauce, 98
Avocado, and Black Bean Salad, Chili Tofu, 50

B

Bananas Foster Sundaes, 114
Barbecue Tofu Bowl, Spicy Korean-Inspired, 70–71
Beans
  Black Bean and Sweet Potato Enchiladas, 75
  Chili Tofu, Avocado, and Black Bean Salad, 50
  Chipotle Sweet Potato and Navy Bean Stew, 73
  Italian-Style Zucchini, Spinach, and Bean Skillet, 65
  Mediterranean-Inspired White Bean and Olive Pasta Salad, 87
  Mixed Bean and Corn Salad, 51
  Spicy Mixed Bean Jambalaya, 80
  Sun-Dried Tomato and White Bean Hummus Flatbreads, 33
Berries
  Blueberry Lemon Pancakes, 26

Mixed Berry Breakfast Bread Pudding, 25
Raspberry PB&J Muffins, 36
Bowls
  Spicy Korean-Inspired Barbecue Tofu Bowl, 70–71
  Tex-Mex Polenta Bowl, 72
Bread Pudding, Mixed Berry Breakfast, 25
Breakfast and brunch
  Blueberry Lemon Pancakes, 26
  Chocolate Orange French Toast, 27
  Creamy Spinach and Mushroom Oatmeal, 23
  Loaded Breakfast Sweet Potatoes, 24
  Maple Quinoa Fruit Salad, 18
  Mixed Berry Breakfast Bread Pudding, 25
  Sun-Dried Tomato and Zucchini Scones, 20
  Tempeh Hash-Stuffed Portobellos, 22
  Tomato and Almond Ricotta Toasts, 21
  Turkish-Style Chickpea Cilbir, 19
Broccoli, 15-Minute White Mac and "Cheese" with, 100
Bruschetta Spaghetti, 85
Buffalo Smashed Chickpea Sandwich, 56
Butter Chicken Sauce and Cherry Tomatoes, Fusilli with, 99

C

Cabbage Rolls, Unstuffed, 81
Carrot Cake Energy Bites, 105
Cashews, Ginger Coconut Tofu with Snap Peas and, 67
Cauliflower Wings, Spicy Tahini, 32
Cherry Cheesecake Jars, 115
Chickpeas
  Baked Chickpea "Chick'n" Nuggets, 37
  Buffalo Smashed Chickpea Sandwich, 56
  Easy Lahmajoun (Armenian-Style Pizza), 64
  Middle Eastern–Inspired Chopped Chickpea Salad, 52
  Not-Tuna Melt, 54–55
  Pasta e Ceci (Italian-Style Chickpea and Pasta Stew), 94–95
  Turkish-Style Chickpea Cilbir, 19
Chili Tofu, Avocado, and Black Bean Salad, 50
Chipotle Peanut Sesame Salsa, 31
Chipotle Sweet Potato and Navy Bean Stew, 73
Chocolate
  Bakery-Style Giant Chocolate Chip Cookies, 106–107
  Chocolate Espresso Glazed Donuts, 110–111
  Chocolate Orange French Toast, 27
  Maple Chocolate Hazelnut Mousse, 109

Coconut
  Coconut Macaroons, 104
  Ginger Coconut Tofu
      with Snap Peas and
      Cashews, 67
  Pumpkin Coconut Soup, 45
Cookies
  Bakery-Style Giant Chocolate
      Chip Cookies, 106–107
  Coconut Macaroons, 104
  Whipped Shortbread
      Cookies, 108
Corn
  Mixed Bean and Corn
      Salad, 51
  Speedy Potato Corn
      Chowder, 48
Crostini, Smoked
    "Salmon," 34–35
Curry
  Curried Vegetable
      Pad Thai, 89
  Fiery Curry Pasta Salad, 53

D

Desserts
  Apricot Peach Crisp, 113
  Bakery-Style Giant Chocolate
      Chip Cookies, 106–107
  Bananas Foster Sundaes, 114
  Carrot Cake Energy Bites, 105
  Cherry Cheesecake Jars, 115
  Chocolate Espresso Glazed
      Donuts, 110–111
  Coconut Macaroons, 104
  Grapefruit, Lime, and Mint
      Yogurt Parfait, 112
  Maple Chocolate Hazelnut
      Mousse, 109
  Whipped Shortbread
      Cookies, 108
  Donuts, Chocolate Espresso
      Glazed, 110–111

E

Edamame
  Edamame Noodle Salad, 84
  Sweet Chili Edamame, 30
Eggplant, Penne
    Arrabbiata, 90–91
Enchiladas, Black Bean and
    Sweet Potato, 75
Espresso Glazed Donuts,
    Chocolate, 110–111
Everything Bagel Crusted
    Tofu Fillets and Green
    Beans, 68–69

F

Freezer-friendly
  Apricot Peach Crisp, 113
  Baked Chickpea "Chick'n"
      Nuggets, 37
  Golden Gazpacho, 44
  Mediterranean-Inspired
      Red Lentil Soup, 47
  Pasta e Ceci (Italian-Style
      Chickpea and Pasta
      Stew), 94–95
  Pumpkin Coconut Soup, 45
  Speedy Potato Corn
      Chowder, 48
  Spicy Mixed Bean
      Jambalaya, 80
  Tortilla Soup, 46
French Toast, Chocolate
    Orange, 27
Fruit Salad, Maple Quinoa, 18

G

Garlic Bread Pinwheels,
    Pepperoncini and
    Roasted Red Pepper, 38
Ginger Coconut Tofu with
    Snap Peas and
    Cashews, 67
Gluten-free

Baked Chickpea "Chick'n"
    Nuggets, 37
Bananas Foster Sundaes, 114
Carrot Cake Energy
    Bites, 105
Chili Tofu, Avocado, and
    Black Bean Salad, 50
Chipotle Peanut
    Sesame Salsa, 31
Chipotle Sweet Potato and
    Navy Bean Stew, 73
Coconut Macaroons, 104
Curried Vegetable
    Pad Thai, 89
Everything Bagel Crusted
    Tofu Fillets and Green
    Beans, 68–69
Ginger Coconut Tofu
    with Snap Peas and
    Cashews, 67
Golden Gazpacho, 44
Grapefruit, Lime, and Mint
    Yogurt Parfait, 112
Italian-Style Zucchini, Spinach,
    and Bean Skillet, 65
Japchae (Korean-Style
    Mixed Vegetables and
    Glass Noodles), 86
Jeweled Rice, 66
Lemon Quinoa Artichoke
    Salad, 49
Loaded Breakfast Sweet
    Potatoes, 24
Maple Chocolate Hazelnut
    Mousse, 109
Maple Quinoa Fruit
    Salad, 18
Mediterranean-Inspired
    Red Lentil Soup, 47
Middle Eastern–Inspired
    Chopped Chickpea
    Salad, 52
Mixed Bean and Corn
    Salad, 51

Moo Shu Lettuce Cups, 39
Polenta-Stuffed Portobello
    Stacks, 78
Portobello-Steak Tacos, 74
Pumpkin Coconut Soup, 45
Spicy Korean-Inspired
    Barbecue Tofu
    Bowl, 70–71
Spicy Mixed Bean
    Jambalaya, 80
Spicy Sesame Broad
    Rice Noodles, 92
Spicy Tahini Cauliflower
    Wings, 32
Sweet Chili Edamame, 30
Tempeh and Asian
    Pear Bulgogi, 79
Tempeh Hash-Stuffed
    Portobellos, 22
Tex-Mex Polenta Bowl, 72
Tortilla Soup, 46
Tteokbokki (Spicy
    Korean-Style Rice
    Cake Stew), 76–77
Unstuffed Cabbage Rolls, 81
Grapefruit, Lime, and Mint
    Yogurt Parfait, 112
Green Beans, Everything
    Bagel Crusted Tofu
    Fillets and, 68–69
Grocery shopping, 13

H

Hazelnut Mousse, Maple
    Chocolate, 109
Hummus Flatbreads,
    Sun-Dried Tomato
    and White Bean, 33

I

Ingredient staples, 10–11

J

Jackfruit Wraps, Jerk, 57
Japchae (Korean-Style
    Mixed Vegetables and
    Glass Noodles), 86

L

Lemons
    Blueberry Lemon
        Pancakes, 26
    Lemon Mushroom Orzo with
        Spinach and Peas, 93
    Lemon Quinoa Artichoke
        Salad, 49
    Linguini with Artichokes in
        Lemon Dill Sauce, 98
Lentil Soup, Mediterranean-
    Inspired Red, 47
Lettuce Cups, Moo Shu, 39
Lime, and Mint Yogurt Parfait,
    Grapefruit, 112

M

Maple syrup
    Maple Chocolate Hazelnut
        Mousse, 109
    Maple Quinoa Fruit Salad, 18
Meal prepping, 5–6
Measuring ingredients, 6
Mint Yogurt Parfait, Grapefruit,
    Lime, and, 112
Moo Shu Lettuce Cups, 39
Muffins, Raspberry PB&J, 36
Mushrooms
    Creamy Spinach and
        Mushroom Oatmeal, 23
    Lemon Mushroom Orzo with
        Spinach and Peas, 93
    Polenta-Stuffed Portobello
        Stacks, 78
    Portobello-Steak Tacos, 74

Tempeh Hash-Stuffed
    Portobellos, 22

N

Nachos, Green Goddess
    Dip, 40–41
Noodles. See Pasta and noodles
Nut-free
    Apricot Peach Crisp, 113
    Bakery-Style Giant Chocolate
        Chip Cookies, 106–107
    Black Bean and Sweet
        Potato Enchiladas, 75
    Blueberry Lemon
        Pancakes, 26
    Bruschetta Spaghetti, 85
    Buffalo Smashed Chickpea
        Sandwich, 56
    Carrot Cake Energy Bites, 105
    Cherry Cheesecake Jars, 115
    Chili Tofu, Avocado, and
        Black Bean Salad, 50
    Chipotle Sweet Potato and
        Navy Bean Stew, 73
    Creamy Pumpkin Penne, 97
    Creamy Spinach and
        Mushroom Oatmeal, 23
    Easy Lahmajoun (Armenian-
        Style Pizza), 64
    Edamame Noodle Salad, 84
    Everything Bagel Crusted
        Tofu Fillets and Green
        Beans, 68–69
    Fiery Curry Pasta Salad, 53
    15-Minute White Mac and
        "Cheese" with Broccoli, 100
    Fusilli with Butter Chicken
        Sauce and Cherry
        Tomatoes, 99
    Golden Gazpacho, 44
    Green Goddess Dip
        Nachos, 40–41

Italian-Style Zucchini, Spinach, and Bean Skillet, 65
Japanese-Style Mixed Vegetable Noodles, 88
Japchae (Korean-Style Mixed Vegetables and Glass Noodles), 86
Jerk Jackfruit Wraps, 57
Lemon Mushroom Orzo with Spinach and Peas, 93
Lemon Quinoa Artichoke Salad, 49
Linguini with Artichokes in Lemon Dill Sauce, 98
Loaded Breakfast Sweet Potatoes, 24
Maple Quinoa Fruit Salad, 18
Mediterranean-Inspired Red Lentil Soup, 47
Mediterranean-Inspired White Bean and Olive Pasta Salad, 87
Middle Eastern–Inspired Chopped Chickpea Salad, 52
Mixed Bean and Corn Salad, 51
Moo Shu Lettuce Cups, 39
Nashville Hot Tofu Sandwich, 58–59
Not-Tuna Melt, 54–55
Pasta e Ceci (Italian-Style Chickpea and Pasta Stew), 94–95
Penne Arrabbiata with Eggplant, 90–91
Pepperoncini and Roasted Red Pepper Garlic Bread Pinwheels, 38
Polenta-Stuffed Portobello Stacks, 78
Portobello-Steak Tacos, 74
Pumpkin Coconut Soup, 45

Smoked "Salmon" Crostini, 34–35
Speedy Potato Corn Chowder, 48
Spicy Korean-Inspired Barbecue Tofu Bowl, 70–71
Spicy Mixed Bean Jambalaya, 80
Spicy Sesame Broad Rice Noodles, 92
Spicy Tahini Cauliflower Wings, 32
Sun-Dried Tomato and Roasted Red Pepper Fettuccine Alfredo, 96
Sun-Dried Tomato and White Bean Hummus Flatbreads, 33
Sun-Dried Tomato and Zucchini Scones, 20
Sweet Chili Edamame, 30
Tempeh and Asian Pear Bulgogi, 79
Tempeh Hash-Stuffed Portobellos, 22
Tex-Mex Polenta Bowl, 72
Tortilla Soup, 46
Tteokbokki (Spicy Korean-Style Rice Cake Stew), 76–77
Turkish-Style Chickpea Cilbir, 19
Un-Crab Salad Po' Boy, 60
Unstuffed Cabbage Rolls, 81
Whipped Shortbread Cookies, 108

O

Oatmeal, Creamy Spinach and Mushroom, 23
Oil-free, 4, 15
    Baked Chickpea "Chick'n" Nuggets, 37

Black Bean and Sweet Potato Enchiladas, 75
Bruschetta Spaghetti, 85
Buffalo Smashed Chickpea Sandwich, 56
Carrot Cake Energy Bites, 105
Chili Tofu, Avocado, and Black Bean Salad, 50
Chipotle Peanut Sesame Salsa, 31
Chipotle Sweet Potato and Navy Bean Stew, 73
Coconut Macaroons, 104
Creamy Pumpkin Penne, 97
Creamy Spinach and Mushroom Oatmeal, 23
Easy Lahmajoun (Armenian-Style Pizza), 64
Edamame Noodle Salad, 84
Everything Bagel Crusted Tofu Fillets and Green Beans, 68–69
15-Minute White Mac and "Cheese" with Broccoli, 100
Ginger Coconut Tofu with Snap Peas and Cashews, 67
Grapefruit, Lime, and Mint Yogurt Parfait, 112
Italian-Style Zucchini, Spinach, and Bean Skillet, 65
Japanese-Style Mixed Vegetable Noodles, 88
Jerk Jackfruit Wraps, 57
Loaded Breakfast Sweet Potatoes, 24
Maple Quinoa Fruit Salad, 18
Mixed Berry Breakfast Bread Pudding, 25
Not-Tuna Melt, 54–55
Polenta-Stuffed Portobello Stacks, 78
Raspberry PB&J Muffins, 36

Nut-free (*continued*)
  Smoked "Salmon"
    Crostini, 34–35
  Spicy Mixed Bean
    Jambalaya, 80
  Spicy Sesame Broad
    Rice Noodles, 92
  Spicy Tahini Cauliflower
    Wings, 32
  Sun-Dried Tomato and
    Roasted Red Pepper
    Fettuccine Alfredo, 96
  Sun-Dried Tomato and
    White Bean Hummus
    Flatbreads, 33
  Tex-Mex Polenta Bowl, 72
  Tomato and Almond
    Ricotta Toasts, 21
  Unstuffed Cabbage
    Rolls, 81
Olive Pasta Salad,
    Mediterranean-Inspired
    White Bean and, 87
One-pot
  Bananas Foster Sundaes, 114
  Black Bean and Sweet
    Potato Enchiladas, 75
  Carrot Cake Energy Bites, 105
  Chipotle Sweet Potato and
    Navy Bean Stew, 73
  Creamy Spinach and
    Mushroom Oatmeal, 23
  Golden Gazpacho, 44
  Grapefruit, Lime, and Mint
    Yogurt Parfait, 112
  Green Goddess Dip
    Nachos, 40–41
  Italian-Style Zucchini, Spinach,
    and Bean Skillet, 65
  Japanese-Style Mixed
    Vegetable Noodles, 88
  Jerk Jackfruit Wraps, 57

Loaded Breakfast Sweet
  Potatoes, 24
Mediterranean-Inspired
  Red Lentil Soup, 47
Mixed Berry Breakfast
  Bread Pudding, 25
Moo Shu Lettuce Cups, 39
Pasta e Ceci (Italian-Style
  Chickpea and Pasta
  Stew), 94–95
Polenta-Stuffed Portobello
  Stacks, 78
Speedy Potato Corn
  Chowder, 48
Spicy Mixed Bean
  Jambalaya, 80
Sweet Chili Edamame, 30
Tomato and Almond
  Ricotta Toasts, 21
Tortilla Soup, 46
Orange French Toast,
  Chocolate, 27

P

Pad Thai, Curried Vegetable, 89
Pancakes, Blueberry Lemon, 26
Pasta and noodles
  Bruschetta Spaghetti, 85
  Creamy Pumpkin Penne, 97
  Curried Vegetable
    Pad Thai, 89
  Edamame Noodle Salad, 84
  Fiery Curry Pasta Salad, 53
  15-Minute White Mac and
    "Cheese" with Broccoli, 100
  Fusilli with Butter Chicken
    Sauce and Cherry
    Tomatoes, 99
  Japanese-Style Mixed
    Vegetable Noodles, 88
  Japchae (Korean-Style
    Mixed Vegetables and
    Glass Noodles), 86

Lemon Mushroom Orzo with
  Spinach and Peas, 93
Linguini with Artichokes in
  Lemon Dill Sauce, 98
Mediterranean-Inspired
  White Bean and Olive
  Pasta Salad, 87
Pasta e Ceci (Italian-Style
  Chickpea and Pasta
  Stew), 94–95
Penne Arrabbiata with
  Eggplant, 90–91
Spicy Sesame Broad
  Rice Noodles, 92
Sun-Dried Tomato and
  Roasted Red Pepper
  Fettuccine Alfredo, 96
Peach Crisp, Apricot, 113
Peanut butter
  Chipotle Peanut
    Sesame Salsa, 31
  Raspberry PB&J Muffins, 36
Pear Bulgogi, Tempeh
  and Asian, 79
Peas
  Ginger Coconut Tofu
    with Snap Peas and
    Cashews, 67
  Lemon Mushroom Orzo with
    Spinach and Peas, 93
Peppers
  Pepperoncini and Roasted
    Red Pepper Garlic
    Bread Pinwheels, 38
  Sun-Dried Tomato and
    Roasted Red Pepper
    Fettuccine Alfredo, 96
Pizzas and flatbreads
  Easy Lahmajoun (Armenian-
    Style Pizza), 64
  Sun-Dried Tomato and
    White Bean Hummus
    Flatbreads, 33

Polenta
  Polenta-Stuffed Portobello
    Stacks, 78
  Tex-Mex Polenta Bowl, 72
Potato Corn Chowder,
  Speedy, 48
Pumpkin
  Creamy Pumpkin Penne, 97
  Pumpkin Coconut Soup, 45

Q

Quinoa
  Lemon Quinoa Artichoke
    Salad, 49
  Maple Quinoa Fruit Salad, 18

R

Recipes, about, 9, 13–15
Rice
  Jeweled Rice, 66
  Spicy Mixed Bean
    Jambalaya, 80
  Unstuffed Cabbage Rolls, 81
Rice cakes
  Tteokbokki (Spicy
    Korean-Style Rice
    Cake Stew), 76–77
Ricotta Toasts, Tomato
  and Almond, 21

S

Salads
  Chili Tofu, Avocado, and
    Black Bean Salad, 50
  Edamame Noodle Salad, 84
  Fiery Curry Pasta Salad, 53
  Lemon Quinoa Artichoke
    Salad, 49
  Mediterranean-Inspired
    White Bean and Olive
    Pasta Salad, 87
  Middle Eastern–Inspired
    Chopped Chickpea
    Salad, 52

Mixed Bean and Corn
  Salad, 51
Salsa, Chipotle Peanut
  Sesame, 31
Salt-free cooking, 15
Sandwiches and wraps
  Buffalo Smashed Chickpea
    Sandwich, 56
  Jerk Jackfruit Wraps, 57
  Nashville Hot Tofu
    Sandwich, 58–59
  Not-Tuna Melt, 54–55
  Un-Crab Salad Po' Boy, 60
Scones, Sun-Dried Tomato
  and Zucchini, 20
Seasoning blends, 7
Sesame Broad Rice
  Noodles, Spicy, 92
Snacks
  Baked Chickpea "Chick'n"
    Nuggets, 37
  Chipotle Peanut
    Sesame Salsa, 31
  Green Goddess Dip
    Nachos, 40–41
  Moo Shu Lettuce Cups, 39
  Pepperoncini and Roasted
    Red Pepper Garlic
    Bread Pinwheels, 38
  Raspberry PB&J Muffins, 36
  Smoked "Salmon"
    Crostini, 34–35
  Spicy Tahini Cauliflower
    Wings, 32
  Sun-Dried Tomato and
    White Bean Hummus
    Flatbreads, 33
  Sweet Chili Edamame, 30
Soups and stews
  Chipotle Sweet Potato and
    Navy Bean Stew, 73
  Golden Gazpacho, 44
  Mediterranean-Inspired
    Red Lentil Soup, 47

Pasta e Ceci (Italian-Style
  Chickpea and Pasta
  Stew), 94–95
Pumpkin Coconut Soup, 45
Speedy Potato Corn
  Chowder, 48
Spicy Mixed Bean
  Jambalaya, 80
Tortilla Soup, 46
Tteokbokki (Spicy
  Korean-Style Rice
  Cake Stew), 76–77
Soy-free
  Apricot Peach Crisp, 113
  Baked Chickpea "Chick'n"
    Nuggets, 37
  Bakery-Style Giant Chocolate
    Chip Cookies, 106–107
  Bananas Foster Sundaes, 114
  Black Bean and Sweet
    Potato Enchiladas, 75
  Bruschetta Spaghetti, 85
  Buffalo Smashed Chickpea
    Sandwich, 56
  Carrot Cake Energy
    Bites, 105
  Cherry Cheesecake Jars, 115
  Chipotle Peanut
    Sesame Salsa, 31
  Chipotle Sweet Potato and
    Navy Bean Stew, 73
  Chocolate Espresso Glazed
    Donuts, 110–111
  Chocolate Orange
    French Toast, 27
  Coconut Macaroons, 104
  Creamy Pumpkin Penne, 97
  Creamy Spinach and
    Mushroom Oatmeal, 23
  Easy Lahmajoun (Armenian-
    Style Pizza), 64
  Fiery Curry Pasta Salad, 53

Fusilli with Butter Chicken Sauce and Cherry Tomatoes, 99
Golden Gazpacho, 44
Grapefruit, Lime, and Mint Yogurt Parfait, 112
Green Goddess Dip Nachos, 40–41
Italian-Style Zucchini, Spinach, and Bean Skillet, 65
Jerk Jackfruit Wraps, 57
Jeweled Rice, 66
Lemon Mushroom Orzo with Spinach and Peas, 93
Lemon Quinoa Artichoke Salad, 49
Linguini with Artichokes in Lemon Dill Sauce, 98
Loaded Breakfast Sweet Potatoes, 24
Maple Quinoa Fruit Salad, 18
Mediterranean-Inspired Red Lentil Soup, 47
Mediterranean-Inspired White Bean and Olive Pasta Salad, 87
Middle Eastern–Inspired Chopped Chickpea Salad, 52
Mixed Bean and Corn Salad, 51
Mixed Berry Breakfast Bread Pudding, 25
Pasta e Ceci (Italian-Style Chickpea and Pasta Stew), 94–95
Penne Arrabbiata with Eggplant, 90–91
Pepperoncini and Roasted Red Pepper Garlic Bread Pinwheels, 38

Polenta-Stuffed Portobello Stacks, 78
Pumpkin Coconut Soup, 45
Raspberry PB&J Muffins, 36
Spicy Mixed Bean Jambalaya, 80
Spicy Tahini Cauliflower Wings, 32
Sun-Dried Tomato and Roasted Red Pepper Fettuccine Alfredo, 96
Sun-Dried Tomato and White Bean Hummus Flatbreads, 33
Tempeh Hash-Stuffed Portobellos, 22
Tex-Mex Polenta Bowl, 72
Tomato and Almond Ricotta Toasts, 21
Tortilla Soup, 46
Turkish-Style Chickpea Cilbir, 19
Whipped Shortbread Cookies, 108
Spinach
Creamy Spinach and Mushroom Oatmeal, 23
Italian-Style Zucchini, Spinach, and Bean Skillet, 65
Lemon Mushroom Orzo with Spinach and Peas, 93
Sundaes, Bananas Foster, 114
Sun-Dried Tomato and White Bean Hummus Flatbreads, 33
Sweet potatoes
Black Bean and Sweet Potato Enchiladas, 75

Chipotle Sweet Potato and Navy Bean Stew, 73
Loaded Breakfast Sweet Potatoes, 24

T
Tacos, Portobello-Steak, 74
Tahini Cauliflower Wings, Spicy, 32
Tempeh
Tempeh and Asian Pear Bulgogi, 79
Tempeh Hash-Stuffed Portobellos, 22
Time-saving strategies, 7–8
Toasts, Tomato and Almond Ricotta, 21
Tofu
Chili Tofu, Avocado, and Black Bean Salad, 50
Everything Bagel Crusted Tofu Fillets and Green Beans, 68–69
Ginger Coconut Tofu with Snap Peas and Cashews, 67
Maple Chocolate Hazelnut Mousse, 109
Nashville Hot Tofu Sandwich, 58–59
Spicy Korean-Inspired Barbecue Tofu Bowl, 70–71
Un-Crab Salad Po' Boy, 60
Tomatoes
Bruschetta Spaghetti, 85
Chipotle Peanut Sesame Salsa, 31
Fusilli with Butter Chicken Sauce and Cherry Tomatoes, 99
Penne Arrabbiata with Eggplant, 90–91
Tomatoes (continued)

Sun-Dried Tomato and
Roasted Red Pepper
Fettuccine Alfredo, 96
Sun-Dried Tomato and
White Bean Hummus
Flatbreads, 33
Sun-Dried Tomato and
Zucchini Scones, 20
Tomato and Almond
Ricotta Toasts, 21
Tools and equipment, 11–12
Tortilla Soup, 46
Tteokbokki (Spicy Korean-Style
Rice Cake Stew), 76–77

V

Vegan diets, 1–4
Vegetables. *See also specific*
Curried Vegetable
Pad Thai, 89
Japanese-Style Mixed
Vegetable Noodles, 88
Japchae (Korean-Style
Mixed Vegetables and
Glass Noodles), 86

Y

Yogurt Parfait, Grapefruit,
Lime, and Mint, 112

Z

Zucchini
Italian-Style Zucchini,
Spinach, and Bean
Skillet, 65
Sun-Dried Tomato and
Zucchini Scones, 20

ACKNOWLEDGMENTS

Creating a cookbook takes the dedication and hard work of a large team of people all pushing toward the same goal. I'm grateful for the opportunity to again work with such an amazing team at Callisto Media to bring this book to life.

A big thank-you to Vanessa Putt for giving me the opportunity to write this book; to my editor, Rachelle Cihonski, who embarked on this journey with me and helped build this manuscript into a successful finished book. Thanks for all your inspiring words, enthusiasm, and guidance—and for always graciously answering all my millions of questions!

To my development editor, Beth Adelman, thank you for ensuring this book "works" and making my recipes come to life. To the entire production, art, and marketing teams assigned to this project—thank you for all your hard work to build and promote this book. Your work is truly appreciated.

ABOUT THE AUTHOR

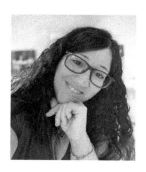

Ally Lazare is a Toronto-based writer and home cook. She is the author of four vegan cookbooks: *Ally's Kitchen: Comfort Food*; *The Budget-Friendly Vegan Cookbook*; *Vegan Dessert Cookbook*; and *Plant-Based Diet in 30 Minutes*.

Ally has been creating recipes since her teenage years and has spent the past decade developing easy, healthy, and delicious plant-based dishes that everyone can enjoy. Ally shares these vegan culinary adventures with others through social media and on her blog.

When she's not cooking, Ally is busy collecting vintage cookbooks and spending time with her husband and two young daughters. You can follow Ally's culinary journeys on Instagram at @allylazare.

CPSIA information can be obtained
at www.ICGtesting.com
Printed in the USA
JSHW010257040122
21706JS00002B/2